Metformin - Pharmacology and Drug Interactions

Edited by Juber Akhtar, Usama Ahmad, Badruddeen and Mohammad Irfan Khan

Published in London, United Kingdom

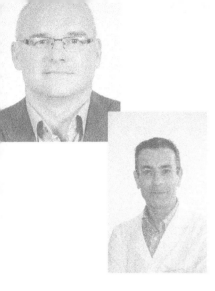
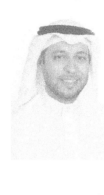
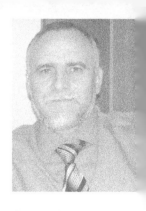
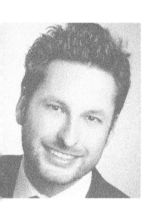
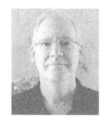
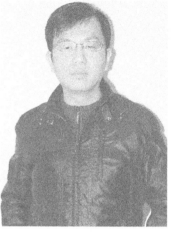

IntechOpen

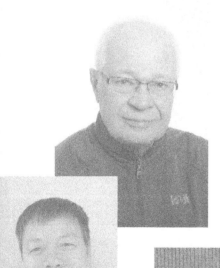
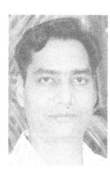
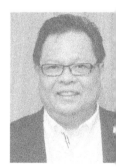
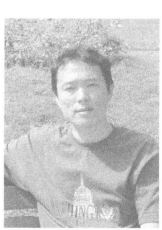
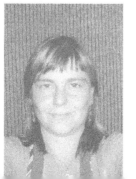

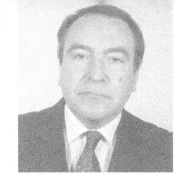
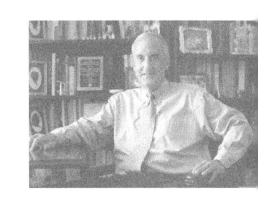
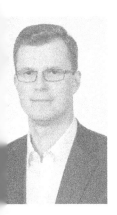
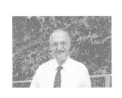
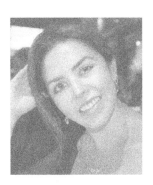

Supporting open minds since 2005

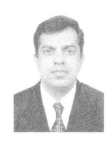
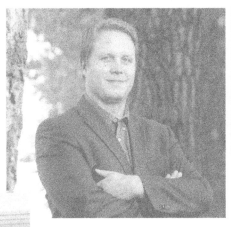
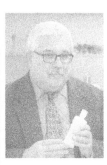
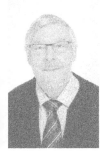
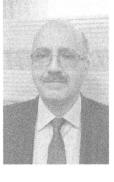
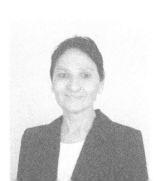
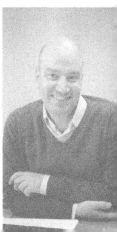

Metformin - Pharmacology and Drug Interactions
http://dx.doi.org/10.5772/intechopen.94707
Edited by Juber Akhtar, Usama Ahmad, Badruddeen and Mohammad Irfan Khan

Contributors
Bernadette Dian Novita, Ari Christy Mulyono, Ferdinand Erwin, Tadesse Sheleme, Safila Naveed, Halima
Sadia, Shalini Sivadasan, Rajasekaran Aiyalu, Muthukumar Subramanian, Sabu Mandumpal Chacko, Priya
Thambi Thekkekara, Samira Abdulla Mahmood, Lucy A. Ochola, Eric M. Guantai

Notice
Statements and opinions expressed in the chapters are these of the individual contributors and not
necessarily those of the editors or publisher. No responsibility is accepted for the accuracy of
information contained in the published chapters. The publisher assumes no responsibility for any
damage or injury to persons or property arising out of the use of any materials, instructions, methods
or ideas contained in the book.

First published in London, United Kingdom, 2021 by IntechOpen
IntechOpen is the global imprint of INTECHOPEN LIMITED, registered in England and Wales,
registration number: 11086078, 5 Princes Gate Court, London, SW7 2QJ, United Kingdom
Printed in Croatia

British Library Cataloguing-in-Publication Data
A catalogue record for this book is available from the British Library

Additional hard and PDF copies can be obtained from orders@intechopen.com

Metformin - Pharmacology and Drug Interactions
Edited by Juber Akhtar, Usama Ahmad, Badruddeen and Mohammad Irfan Khan
p. cm.
Print ISBN 978-1-83969-605-3
Online ISBN 978-1-83969-606-0
eBook (PDF) ISBN 978-1-83969-607-7

Meet the editors

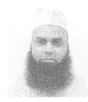 Dr. Juber Akhtar obtained BPharm from Jamia Hamdard University, New Delhi, in 2005, MPharm from Manipal University, Karnataka, in 2007, and Ph.D. from Integral University, Lucknow, in 2014. He is currently employed as an associate professor at Integral University. From 2014 to 2016, Dr. Akhtar was head of the Faculty of Pharmacy, Integral University. He also served as chairman cum biological scientist for Institutional Animal Ethics Committee (IAEC) from October 2015 to May 2017. He has experience teaching abroad and was previously a professor at Buraydah College of Pharmacy and Dentistry, Kingdom of Saudi Arabia (KSA). Dr. Akhtar has more than eighty publications in reputed journals and is an editorial board member for many esteemed journals. He has supervised a dozen Ph.D. and MPharm students in research projects. Dr. Akhtar's areas of research interest include the development of nanoparticulate drug delivery systems.

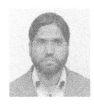 Dr. Badruddeen obtained both a BPharm and MPharm from Hamdard University, Delhi. He obtained a Ph.D. in Pharmacology from Integral University, Lucknow, in 2014. He has expertise in cardiovascular, neurodegenerative, and endocrine diseases. He has fourteen years of experience conducting research on the safety, toxicity, and clinical efficacy of herbal and allopathic drugs. He has sixty-five original articles in reputed journals to his credit. Dr. Badruddeen is also an editorial board member for several journals. He has supervised a dozen research scholars and is member secretary of the Institutional Animal Ethics Committee (IAEC) and in-charge, animal house, Integral University since June 2008.

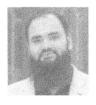 Dr. Usama Ahmad holds a specialization in Pharmaceutics from Amity University, Lucknow, India. He received his Ph.D. degree from Integral University on his work titled 'Development and evaluation of silymarin nanoformulation for hepatic carcinoma'. Currently, he's working as an Assistant Professor of Pharmaceutics in the Faculty of Pharmacy, Integral University. He has been teaching Pharm.D, B.Pharm, and M.Pharm students and conducting research in the novel drug delivery domain. From 2013 to 2014 he worked on a research project funded by SERB-DST, Government of India. He has a rich publication record with more than 24 original articles published in reputed journals, 2 edited books with IntechOpen, 4 book chapters, and a number of scientific articles published in 'Ingredients South Asia Magazine' and 'QualPharma Magazine'. He is a member of the American Association for Cancer Research, International Association for the Study of Lung Cancer, and the British Society for Nanomedicine. Dr. Ahmad's research focus is on the development of nanoformulations to facilitate the delivery of drugs that aim to provide practical solutions to current healthcare problems.

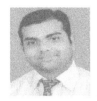 Dr. Mohammad Irfan Khan holds a Bachelor's and Master's degree of Pharmacy from Hamdard University, Delhi. He has a Ph.D. with a specialization in Phytochemistry. He has expertise in Ayurvedic and Nutraceuticals and worked with some of the major Pharmaceutical companies. He has 12 years of experience in the Research & Formulation development of Ayurvedic, Herbal and Nutraceutical products and successfully developed more than 100 formulations. He has more than 38 original papers in international journals of repute. Dr. Khan has also supervised many research scholars at PG and Ph.D. levels.

Contents

Preface

Discovered in 1922, metformin is an oral antidiabetic drug used to control blood sugar levels. It is on the World Health Organization's List of Essential Medicines and is a the first-line treatment for type 2 diabetes, predominantly in people who are overweight. It is a biguanide antihyperglycemic agent that works by decreasing glucose production by the liver, increasing the insulin sensitivity of body tissues, and increasing GDF15 secretion, which reduces appetite and caloric intake.

This book highlights the molecular mechanism, pharmacokinetics, and uses of metformin, as well as presents information on adverse drug reactions, drug interactions, and the potential use of metformin in tuberculosis. Dedicated chapters discuss the mechanism of metformin; its clinical pharmacokinetics, including absorption, distribution, metabolism, and excretion; adverse effects of the medicine, such as diarrhea, nausea, abdominal pain, low blood sugar, elevated blood lactic acid level (caused by overly large doses or occurring in persons with severe kidney problems); and recent advancements in the use of metformin for tuberculosis.

This volume is a useful resource for students, researchers, clinical practitioners, and other interested readers.

Dr. Juber Akhtar
Associate Professor,
Faculty of Pharmacy,
Integral University,
Lucknow, India

Usama Ahmad, Badruddeen and Mohammad Irfan Khan
Integral University,
India

Section 1

Mechanism of Action

Chapter 1

Mechanisms of Action of Metformin

Samira Abdulla Mahmood

Abstract

Metformin is the first-choice drug for treatment of type 2 diabetes notably those associated with obesity. It does not only reduce hyperglycemia, but also possesses pleiotropic effects opening the pave for numerous potential clinical applications. In this chapter we illustrate the various mechanisms of metformin action in reduction of hepatic glucose output, improvement of insulin action, restoration of fat metabolism and gut microbiome, reduction of inflammation, upregulation of antioxidant enzymes, and attenuation of tumor growth. Understanding of such mechanisms might propose further clinical applications for metformin.

Keywords: 5' AMP-activated protein kinase (AMPK), metformin, gluconeogenesis, antioxidant, mammalian target of rapamycin (mTOR), complex 1

1. Introduction

The mechanisms underlying metformin actions appear to be complex and responsible for the pleiotropic effects of metformin. These mechanisms remain a topic of considerable debate. Actually, in the last decade we moved from a simple picture, that metformin acts via the liver 5' AMP-activated protein kinase (AMPK), to a much more complex one, reflecting its various mechanisms in different cells and tissues.

Since the early studies have suggested that metformin acts by inhibition of complex 1 in mitochondrial electron transport chain [1] and subsequently activation of AMPK [2, 3], AMPK-independent targets have also been reported. These comprise dephosphorylation the ribosomal protein S6, suppression of mammalian target of rapamycin complex 1 (mTORC1) activation and signaling via Rag GTPase [4], attenuation of hepatic glucose 6 phosphate levels [5], suppression of redox transfer by mitochondrial glycerophosphate dehydrogenase (mGPD) [6], as well as modulation of inflammation/oxidative stress and oncogenic signaling pathways.

2. Primary molecular mechanism

Metformin, a hydrophilic drug with Pka 12.4, cannot readily be diffuse passively through the cell membrane due to its existence as cation (ionized) at physiological pH 7.4 [7]. As hydrophilic drug it needs a carrier mediated pathway to efficiently pass through the cell membrane. This is facilitated by the organic cation transporter

1(OCT 1) [8], a member of the soluble carrier family 22 (SLC22) of membrane proteins. OCT1 is mostly expressed in the liver for transferring of cations including metformin, but also facilitates the uptake of metformin from the gut lumen to the interstitium [9]. Cells express OCT1 are able to facilitate cellular uptake of metformin which is in consistence with its accumulation in particular targeted organelles. Also, other types of OCT proteins are present at apical or basolateral sites with different functions.

Within the mitochondria metformin accumulates in the matrix and inhibits complex1 electron transfer chain NADH ubiquitin oxidoreductase (NADH) [1, 10, 11], which promotes proton generation. This inhibition reduces NADH oxidation and ultimately prevents ATP production from ATP synthase. By this way, the ratios of AMP: ATP and ADP: ATP increase, **Figure 1**. Increment in these ratios, which accompanied with reduction in cellular energy activates the cellular energy sensor (house keeper enzyme) AMPK [11]. Another consequence of complex 1 inhibition is the higher levels of AMP, which in turn induces AMPK-independent effects. Moreover, metformin directly inhibits hepatic GPD2, the enzyme involves in substrate (glycerol) gluconeogenesis. Its inhibition by metformin leads to increase cytosolic redox and suppression of gluconeogenesis [12].

AMPK is a heterotrimeric protein complex that consists of α, β, and γ sub-units. The α subunit represents the catalytic site that can be activated (phosphorylated) by liver kinase B1 (LKB1) [13] at Thr-172 [14] and also by calcium/ calmodulin-dependent protein kinase kinase β (CaMKKβ) at Thr-172 [15]. The β and γ denote regulatory subunits. In mammals, the γ subunits contain nucleotide-binding sites for AMP or ATP [16]. In case of cellular energy stress with low ATP, AMP or ADP directly and mutually bind to the γ subunits causing conformational change leading to AMPK activation. Metformin induces activation of AMPK by LBK1 pathway and also by AMP/ADP induced conformational changes, too. It is worth to mention that higher levels of AMP protect AMPK from dephosphorylation by phosphatases [17]. AMPK plays a role in several cellular events, including glucose metabolism, lipid metabolism, redox regulation, anti-aging and anti-inflammation [18, 19].

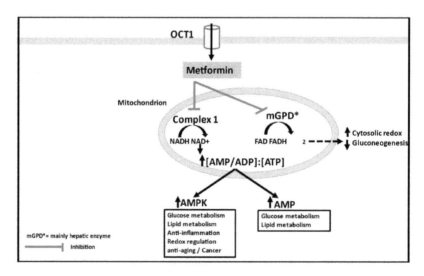

Figure 1.
Primary molecular mechanism of metformin action. For explanation see text.

3. Antihyperglycemic mechanisms of action

Metformin is currently the drug of choice in treating patients with type 2 diabetes mellitus (T2DM). Its mechanisms are still elusive. Nevertheless, it lowers blood glucose through multiple mechanisms. First, it inhibits intestinal absorption of glucose. Second, it suppresses glucose production by the liver. Third, it facilitates glucose uptake into tissues, thus reducing blood glucose levels enabling better health to pancreatic beta-cells. Finally, it improves insulin sensitivity and inflammation. The most accepted action of metformin in T2DM is inhibition of gluconeogenesis and reduction in hepatic glucose output (HGO).

3.1 Mechanisms to lower hepatic gluconeogenesis

Metformin is taken up into the hepatocyte via the OTC1 [20]. Due to the difference in hepatocyte pH and pka of metformin, the drug becomes ionized and positively charge and accumulates in the cells and, further, in the mitochondria to concentrations up to 1000-fold higher than in the extracellular medium [21]. The uptake of positively charge metformin into the mitochondria is derived by the membrane potentials across the plasma membrane and mitochondrial inner membrane (positive outside) [1], Within the mitochondria, metformin inhibits complex1, which reduces ATP production and increases AMP and ADP levels. One consequence of respiratory chain inhibition is increment in ADP:ATP ratios that modestly suppress gluconeogenesis as seen experimentally in cells carrying this process [22], and hinder the hepatocytes from synthetizing the high energy requiring gluconeogenesis [23], **Figure 2**. Other consequence is changes in NAD$^+$:NADH ratios involving in a negative impact on gluconeogenesis [10].

Criticized comments on this mechanism are based on the higher concentration (in millimole levels) on metformin required for rapid complex 1 inhibition, although experimentation in in vitro studies have shown that inhibition of comlpex1 in rat hepatoma (H4IIE) cells does occur at lower concentrations ((50–100 μmol/l)) after long periods due to a slow transport of metformin across mitochondrial membrane [1]. This observation has been confirmed experimentally [24].

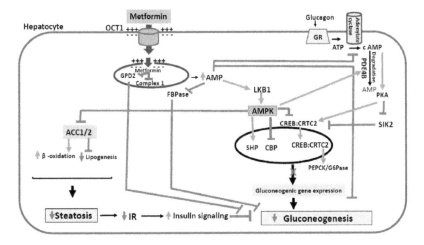

Figure 2.
Mechanism of lowering hepatic gluconeogenesis by metformin (see text).

3.2 Activation of hepatic AMPK

Metformin induced reduction in cellular energy and increment in AMP:ATP ratios are indicative for activation of the energy sensor AMPK by LKB1 (see primary mechanism). Stimulation of AMPK results in repression of anabolism (fatty acid and cholesterol synthesis, gluconeogenesis) and switching on catabolism (fatty acid uptake and oxidation, glucose uptake) [25] in order to restore cell energy hemostasis and prevent cells from damage [26]. The first observation of involvement of AMPK in metformin action was reported in vitro of rat hepatocytes and rat liver in vivo [27]. Moreover, AMPK can also be activated by glucose starvation, exercise and metformin activated lysosomal mechanisms [28].

3.3 AMPK dependent mechanisms

Activated AMPK phosphorylates the cAMP specific 3′,5′-cyclic phosphodiesterase 4B (PDE4B) and activates cAMP degradation (↓cAMP) [21]. Consequently, it prevents the activation of cAMP-dependent protein kinase A (PKA), the enzyme that phosphorylates the transcription factor cAMP response element binding protein (CREB), and then activates CREB-CBP-CRTC2 (CREB:CRTC2) transcription complex involving in transcription of the genes encoding the gluconeogenic enzymes phosphoenolpyruvate carboxykinase (PEPCK) and Glucose 6-phosphatase (G6Pase) [29], **Figure 2**. On the other hand, AMPK induces phosphorylation of CREB binding protein (CBP) at serine 436 leading to dissociation of the CREB-CBP-CRTC2 transcription complex, thus repression of PEPCK and G6Pase [29]. In addition, AMPK or salt-inducible kinase 2 (SIK2) phosphorylates CREB-regulated transcriptional coactivator-2 (CRTC2), thus, inhibits its nuclear translocation and retains in cytoplasm [30]. Moreover, AMPK upregulates the orphan nuclear receptor small heterodimer partner (SHP), that functions as transcription repressor [31] through competition with CRTC2 binding in CREB–CBP complex, **Figure 2**.

Another mechanism mediated by AMPK is inhibition of fat biosynthesis and activation of fat beta-oxidation, resulting in long term enhancement of hepatic insulin sensitivity, which is clinically relevant. Metformin-induced hepatic AMPK phosphorylates the isomers of acetyl-CoA carboxylase (ACC1/ACC2) at serine residues responsible for fat beta-oxidation [32]. Phosphorylation of ACC1 and ACC2 inhibit the conversion of acetyl-CoA to malonyl-CoA resulting in reduction of liver lipogenesis and hepatosteatosis (fatty liver) and increment in fatty acids oxidation, which are factors contributing in improvement of insulin sensitivity/signaling and hyperglycemia. Likewise, activation of AMPK suppresses the expression of lipogenic genes by direct phosphorylation of transcription factors including carbohydrate response element binding protein (ChREBP), **Figure 2**, and by this means regresses the lipogenesis [33], **Figure 2**. Taken together, the role of AMPK involves in phosphorylation of key metabolic enzymes and transcription co-activators/factors modulating gene expression leading to inhibition of glucose, proteins and lipid synthesis and stimulation of glucose uptake and fatty acid oxidation.

3.4 AMPK independent mechanisms

Metformin induced a rise in AMP levels inhibits gluconeogenesis independent of AMPK. AMP allosterically inhibits fructose-1,6-bisphosphatase, a key enzyme of gluconeogenesis and AMP sensitive [34]. This action might be responsible for acute metformin action. In addition, AMP inhibits adenylate cyclase producing cAMP in response to glucagon released in starvation leading to lowering cAMP and reducing expression of gluconeogenesis enzymes [35], **Figure 2**.

Recent proposed mechanism of increased hepatic gluconeogenesis is related to impaired white adipose tissue lipolysis with resultant increase in hepatic uptake of non-esterified fatty acids (NEFA). Hepatic beta-oxidation of NEFA can produce acetyl-coenzyme A (acetyl-CoA), the allosteric activator of the enzyme pyruvate carboxylase that is implicated in the first step f gluconeogenesis by supplying oxaloacetate [36]. Insulin regulates lipolysis of white adipose tissue, thereby, indirectly regulates hepatic gluconeogenesis [37]. Insulin resistance with inflammation in white adipose tissue increases glycerol turnover. Thus, metformin improves insulin sensitivity and reduces resistance leading to suppression of gluconeogenesis.

In addition, white adipose tissue delivers glycerol to the liver. In the liver, glycerol is phosphorylated. Through mitochondrial glycerol-3-phosphate dehydrogenase (GPD2), glycerol is converted into dihydroxyacetone phosphate (DHAP), a component included in gluconeogenesis.

Metformin inhibits GPD2, leading to suppression of DHAP and subsequently gluconeogenesis in substrate (glycerol) specific manner [12]. In context of obesity and T2DM, inhibition of gluconeogenesis from increased supply of glycerol due to dysregulation of white adipose tissue may partially benefit uncontrolled type2 diabetic patients with dysregulated white adipose tissue lipolysis [38].

As discussed above, metformin suppresses gluconeogenesis through interactions with regulatory process of gluconeogenesis as shown in inhibition of transcription (downregulation of gluconeogenic genes expression), substrate (suppression of glycerol induced DHAP formation) and increase cytosolic redox **Figure** 2.

3.5 Mechanisms in skeletal muscle

Metformin affects skeletal muscle metabolism by direct and indirect mechanisms. Emphasis has been placed on the metformin's effect to increase insulin-stimulated peripheral glucose uptake and to reduce glucotoxicity, which indirectly improves muscle glucose uptake [12]. Metformin reduces gluconeogenesis and hepatic glucose output leads to reduce blood glucose levels in type 2 patients, which accompanied by improvement in insulin action. Improvement in insulin levels in circulation under metformin treatment attenuates the hyper-insulinemic pressure on insulin receptors (insensitive phosphorylated receptors) leading to upregulation and increase sensitivity of receptors to insulin [39]. Consequently, muscle glucose uptake is indirectly stimulated by metformin due to reduce insulin resistance in skeletal muscle and peripheral tissues.

In skeletal muscle, activation of AMPK by metformin increases proliferator-activated receptor γ coactivator-1α (PGC-1α), which in turn stimulates glucose transporter 4 (GLUT4) gene transcription [40]. This mechanism induces GLUT4 and others mitochondrial genes required for catabolism. In addition, activated AMPK stimulates the translocation of GLUT4 to the plasma membrane and acutely increase skeletal glucose uptake.

Moreover, AMPK induced phosphorylation of acetyl-CoA-carboxylase-2 (ACC-2) results in reduce malonyl-COA, which is the inhibitor of carnitine O-palmitoyltransferase, leading to increase transport of fatty acids into mitochondria. Thus, fatty acid-oxidation is acutely increased. It worth to mention that these mechanisms are regulated by PGC-1 α, which initiates many genes involved in AMPK functions in skeletal muscle [40], **Figure** 3.

3.6 Mechanism in fat tissue

Obesity has been found to be the most crucial factor for insulin resistance (IR). In addition, insulin sensitivity decreases with age. Therefore, glucose entry into

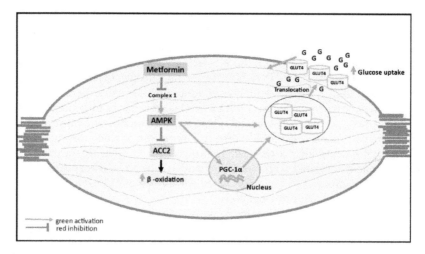

Figure 3.
Mechanism of increase muscle responsiveness by metformin (see text).

tissues, including muscle and fat, decreases, since adipocytes have fewer insulin receptors. Metformin improves lipid profile in patients with T2DM. Insulin resistance (IR) means reduces tissue responsiveness to insulin with resultant elevation in insulin levels (hyperinsulinemia). Beta-cells produce more insulin, but ultimately fail to overcome IR with resultant loss of beta-cell function and development of hyperglycemia. Risk factors for IR are obesity and inactivity.

The signaling pathway connected with IR is phosphatidylinositol-3-kinase/protein kinase B protein (PI3K/PK), which also known as Akt. Akt is also important for translocation of GLUT4 onto the cell membrane surface of muscle and fat cells for glucose entry [41]. Akt inactivation or defect can lead to impairment of membrane transposition of GLUT4, which results in IR accompanied with hyperinsulinemia, hyperglycemia and cardiac impairment [42]. Metformin activates and restores the PI3K/Akt/GLUT4 signaling in rats with type 2 diabetes [43], thereby suppresses IR.

Metformin enhances disposal of blood glucose into skeletal muscle and fat, thus insulin resistance associated with diabetes is overcome. This can be translated into increase storage of glycogen in skeletal muscle, enhancement of fatty acid oxidation and reduced lipogenesis in adipose tissue, which in general reduce the body fat content.

3.7 Mechanisms in the intestine

Beside the liver, the intestine is also considered as an important target for metformin actions. Metformin lowers blood glucose not only through the action in the circulation, targeting the liver and other organs, but also through one in the intestine. The proposed actions are increase in intestinal glucose entry mainly in enterocytes with anaerobic utilization, resulting in reduced net glucose uptake into blood with enhanced lactate production [44, 45], increase in glucagon like peptide-1 (GLP1) levels, increase bile acid pool within the intestine and modulation of microbiome [46].

Activated AMPK phosphorylates the glucose transporter 2 (GLUT2), which then translocated to the apical membrane of intestinal cells, mainly enterocytes, where it promotes glucose uptake into enterocytes [6]. Metformin increases uptake and utilization (anaerobic) of glucose, where subsequently an increase in plasma lactate is resulted. In fact, the intestine and the liver are implicated in metformin-related lactate production. The effect of metformin in intestinal glucose utilization has been shown in positron emission tomography–computed tomography (PET-CT) imaging of patients treated with metformin. This imaging technique uses positron-emitting 18F-fluorodeoxyglucose (^{18}F-FDG), that its intestinal (mainly in the colon) uptake increases in metformin treated patients confirming increase glucose uptake and metabolism in the gut [46].

Metformin inhibits mitochondrial glycerophosphate dehydrogenase, so the conversion of cytosolic pyruvates to lactate is reduced [6], thus, intracellular lactate levels are built up and then released into the plasma. This has been proved in rat studies, where the hepatic portal vein has been shown as the area with the higher peak of plasma lactate concentrations, implicating the intestine as the main site of metformin-associated anerobic glucose utilization and lactate production (estimated by 10% increase in intestinal lactate concentration) [47].

Another intestinal action of metformin directs to GLP-1, which is secreted from L cells distributed throughout the gut but concentrated in the ileum. As reported in mice studies, metformin increases the expression of the precursor proteins (pre-proglucagon and proglucagon) of GLP-1, thus potentially increasing GLP-1 production and secretion [48]. In addition, metformin affects the enzyme degrading GLP-1, dipeptidyl peptidase-4 (DPP4) by mechanisms that are not well clarified [49]. Moreover, stimulation of GLP-1 secretion can occur indirectly, via the bile acid pool alteration by metformin [46]. Metformin activated AMPK directly phosphorylates and represses bile acid sensor, the farnesoid X receptor (FXR), on ileal cells, which results in reduced FXR transcription activity and subsequently reduced sensing and ileal absorption of bile acids [50]. By its turn, the higher level of bile acid pool stimulates bile acid receptors TGR5 on L cells, inducing secretion of GLP-1 [51]. Furthermore, the consequences of reduced bile acid absorption are lower levels of cholesterol in patients taken chronic metformin [52] and diarrhea associated with metformin intolerance due to osmotic effect mediated by increased luminal bile slats levels [53].

The gut microbiome composition has been shown to contribute to the development of obesity and type 2 diabetes, which implicated in a reduction in bacteria producing short chain fatty acids (SCFAs) such as butyrate-producing bacteria and an increase in opportunistic pathogens as shown in type 2 diabetics [54]. SCFAs are considered as important signaling metabolites that impact hepatic gluconeogenesis and fatty acid metabolism [55]. Metformin modulates gut microbiota and increases SCFAs metabolizing bacteria, which lead to suppression of hepatic gluconeogenesis, reduction in FFA release from adipocytes and appetite suppression via incretin [56].

Metformin alters the microbiome composition in mice and humans, where the bacterium Akkermansia muciniphila is increased, accompanied with associated increase in mucin-producing goblet cells as demonstrated in mice model. Akkermansia muciniphila can increase endocannabinoids, which improve the thickness of gut mucous barrier and reduce inflammation [57], and so improve glucose tolerance. On the other hand, an increase in such bacteria by metformin triggers production of short chain fatty acids butyrate and propionate, which results in reduction of hepatic gluconeogenesis, appetite and weight [46]. Taken together, alteration of microbiome composition by metformin can improve metabolic disorders which needed further investigations.

4. Mechanisms of antiinflammatory/antioxidant

Beyond the glucose lowering actions, metformin can directly and indirectly modulate inflammation. Several experimental and clinical studies demonstrated the anti-inflammatory actions of metformin in endothelial cells (EC) and smooth muscle cells (SMC), monocytes, macrophages and other cell types, where it suppresses the main components of inflammation and restores cell functions [58, 59]. Since inflammation is linked to a number of clinical disorders, thus, metformin can possibly interfere with and ameliorate metabolic disorders, cardiovascular diseases, atherosclerosis, obesity cancer and aging. Although the crucial mechanisms are not well elucidated, accepted anti-inflammatory mechanisms of metformin, which are common and implicated in the before mentioned disorders are presented below.

Activation of AMPK by metformin inhibits nuclear factor kappa light-chain-enhancer of activated B-cells (NF-κB) transcription [60]. NF-κB is a transcription regulator implicated in various inflammatory pathways. Metformin induced NF-κB inhibition suppresses inflammatory pathways, proinflammatory cytokines and reactive oxygen species (ROS) production [61]. Likewise, activation of AMPK-phosphatase and the tensin homolog (PTEN) pathway by metformin suppresses phosphoinositide 3-kinase (PI3K)-Akt pathway that activates NF-κB in human vascular SMC. In this way, NF-κB is also inhibited, **Figure 4**. In addition, metformin suppresses Poly [ADP ribose] polymerase 1 (PARP-1), which functions as a coactivator of NF-κB transcription to stimulate pro-inflammatory pathways. Nitric oxide (NO), a mediator of in nerve, immune and CVS is decreased in oxidative stress induced by hyperglycemia. Metformin increases NO via activation of AMPK, which antagonizes inflammation and ROS production [62]. As well, metformin inhibits the differentiation of monocytes to inflammatory macrophages [63] through activation of AMPK, which reduces the phosphorylation of signal transducer and activator of transcription 3(STAT3), **Figure 4**.

Inhibition of NF-κB transcription triggers consequences in different tissues. In macrophages, inhibition of NF-κB activation by metformin can result in reduction of NO, PGE2, and proinflammatory cytokines, such as IL-1β (interleukin-1 β), TNF-α (tumor necrosis factor - α) [64], IL-6 and IL8 (responsible for calling monocytes and adhesion of endothelial cells) [65]. In human adipocyte, metformin induced inhibition of NF-κB pathway leads to suppression of proinflammatory cytokine-induced 11β-HSD1 (11 β -hydroxysteroid dehydrogenase type 1) expression [66]. 11β-HSD1 is elevated in human adipose tissue in obesity and metabolic syndrome, generates active glucocorticoids and is associated with chronic inflammation. Moreover,

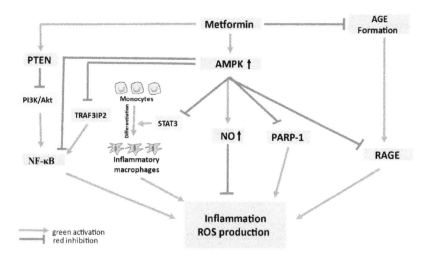

Figure 4.
Potential mechanisms of metformin to attenuate inflammation and production of reactive oxygen species.

inhibition of NF-κB suppresses the expression of CXCL8, a cytokine responsible for changing the microenvironment around the tumor by attracting leukocytes and endothelial progenitors contributed in angiogenesis [67]. Metformin applies its anti-inflammatory action for antifibrotic effect on heart muscle cells through activation of AMPK and inhibition of the pro-inflammatory mediators of the TRAF3 interacting protein (TRAF3IP2) molecule, which induced by aldosterone and enhances production of NF-κB [68]. Furthermore, anti-inflammatory mechanisms associated with atherosclerosis, allergic asthma, hepatic steatosis and vascular injury have been ascribed to metformin but required further elucidations.

In regard of macrophages activity, activated AMPK by metformin reduces phosphorylation of STAT3 (signal transducer and activator of transcription 3), thereby, inhibits the differentiation of monocytes into inflammatory macrophages (M1) [69], while promotes polarization into anti-inflammatory macrophages (M2). These mechanisms place metformin as potential anti-inflammatory targeting macrophages differentiations and polarization with benefits in vascular injury, atherosclerosis, certain cancer and insulin resistance [63].

Further mechanism associated with anti-inflammatory actions of metformin is the inhibition of advance glycation end-products (AGEs) [70], which are one of the crucial inflammatory factor in diabetes, promoting inflammation, ROS production and atherosclerosis [71, 72]. In fact, during hyperglycemia accumulation of glucose in cells facilitates the binding of each two closest glucose molecules with each other to form dicarbonyl compounds, which are percussors of AGEs. AGEs bind to their receptors (RAGE) in different target cells including macrophages, where they promote expression of IL1, IL6, TNF α and RAGE, and activate NF-κB pathway [68], leading to inflammation, apoptosis and fibrotic reactions, as observed in tubular cells. Metformin not only binds chemically to these precursors and renders them inactive, thereby reduces the formation of AGEs, but also suppresses RAGE via activation of AMPK [73]. Altogether, metformin suppresses RAGE/NF-κB pathway, leading to regression of RAGE effects on macrophages and change of their surface markers from inflammatory (M1) to anti-inflammatory (M2) phenotype. **Figure 4** illustrates the potential anti-inflammatory mechanisms of metformin.

Beside the direct effect on proinflammatory pathways, metformin can indirectly reduce inflammation through metabolic consequences. Reduction in hyperglycemia and subsequently the weight as well as the atherogenic LDL cholesterol levels can have favorable effect on chronic inflammation, atherosclerosis and cardiovascular disorders.

As mentioned before, metformin inhibits mitochondrial complex 1 electron transfer complex chain and reduces the production of ROS, which normally formed by synthesis of ATP from ATP synthase. Metformin can reduce ROS through activation of AMPK which inhibits TFG-β, a potent inflammatory factor stimulating the production of ROS and induce endogenous antioxidants such as glutathione reductase (GSH), superoxide dismutase (SOD) and catalase (CAT) [74]. Independent of AMPK activation, metformin can activate antioxidant SOD and clean the damaging effects of ROS in tissues. In addition, it can direct trap hydroxyl peroxide and activate antioxidant enzymes such as catalase, which decomposes H_2O_2. Reduction of ROS reduces IL1β [68]. Therefore, metformin has been shown to play a role in controlling and changing oxidative/inflammatory pathways in clinical and laboratory conditions through various mechanisms.

5. Antineoplastic actions of metformin

The role of metformin in treatment of cancer has been reported in various recent sophisticated publications. Clinical observational studies in liver, colon and pancreatic cancer have demonstrated that metformin prevents and decreases the risk of cancer development [75]. In addition, improvement overall survival outcomes have been reported in patients with colorectal and breast cancer [76], where metformin treated breast cancer patients showed a lower HER-2 positive rate and mortality rate than the control group [77] Besides that, metformin enhances the effects of anti-cancer drugs as shown in vitro and in vivo studies using vincristine, cisplatin, and doxorubicin [78, 79]. Altogether, the results point to involvement of metformin in chemotherapy as adjuvant or a potential anti-cancer candidate which require further experimentations.

Cancer growth and proliferation can be regressed direct and indirect by metformin. Metformin induced reduction in cancer growth has been shown to be indirect through systemic effects related to reduced blood glucose levels, improved insulin resistance and declined pro-inflammatory cytokines. This indirect action might explain the effect of metformin in several types of cancer linked to hyperinsulinemia as a risk factor. Also, metformin directly modulates several oncogenic signaling pathways described in the following text.

As mentioned in different sections of this chapter, the primary mechanism of metformin is to inhibit the oxidative phosphorylation by blockade of complex1 in mitochondria in target cells. Mitochondrial energy reduction and metabolic stress increase the endogenous levels of reactive oxygen species (ROS) which can mediate the death of cancer cells depending on oxidative phosphorylation for gaining energy [24]. Likewise, energy stress seems to hinder cancer cells from synthesis of energy requiring proteins, lipids and structural elements necessary for cancer growth and proliferation. This action can be considered as the first step of metformin induced tumor regression, and growth retardation. Furthermore, deprivation of cancer cells from ATP activates the tumor suppressor gene LKB1 which then phosphorylates AMPK [80] **Figure 5**. AMPK regulates several signaling pathways, primarily via inhibition of mammalian target of rapamycin (mTOR) signaling to suppress tumorigenesis as follows.

Metformin is taken up into cancer cells expressing OCT1, accumulates in mitochondria, blocks complex 1 and activates AMPK. AMPK phosphorylates p53 on ser15 (the tumor suppressor) which is required to start AMPK-dependent cell growth arrest and apoptosis [81], **Figure 5**. On the other hand, activated AMPK

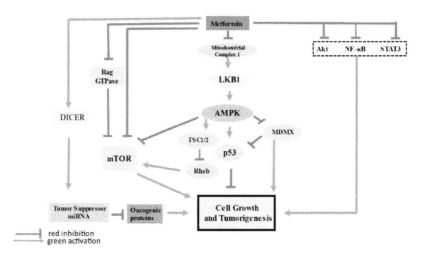

Figure 5.
Mechanisms of metformin suppressing tumorigenesis.

phosphorylates MDMX on ser 367 leading to MDMX inactivation and p53 activation [82]. MDMX and the human MDM2 are partner proteins monitor p53 in a negative feedback fashion and restrain its function to maintain the normal development and function of different tissues [83]. Phosphorylation one of them results in inhibition of ubiquitylation (a molecular change) of p53 leading to stabilization and activation of p53.

Beyond the effect on p53, metformin inhibits mTOR. mTOR is a catalytic subunit, composes of two protein complexes, mTORC1 and mTORC2, that regulate cell growth [84]. Inhibition of mTOR attenuates cell proliferation [85]. Metformin inhibits the activation of mTOR via AMPK-dependent and -independent mechanisms. By AMPK-independent way, metformin phosphorylates directly the regulatory associated protein (raptor) that inactivates mTOR. Likewise, metformin inhibits mTOR signaling by inactivating Rag GTPase [4]. On the other hand, AMPK directly phosphorylates the tumor suppressor tuberous sclerosis complex 2 (TSC2) leading to activation of complex 1 and 2, TSC1/2. TSC1/2 inhibits Rheb, which in turn inactivates mTOR [86] and suppresses cell proliferation.

Besides AMPK and mTOR, metformin has been shown to affect other oncogenic signaling pathways. Metformin suppresses Akt (protein kinase B) expression which is associated with increased phosphatase and tensin (PTEN, a tumor suppressor gene) [87]. This is considered as main mechanism via which endometrial carcinoma is inhibited by metformin. Additionally, metformin inhibits activation of nuclear factor kappa light-chain-enhancer of activated B-cells (NF-κB) and phosphorylation of STAT3 in cancer stem cells [88]. The NF-κB and STAT3 transcription factors are involved in mediating an epigenic switch from non-transformed to cancer cells as shown in breast cancer model. This action suggests that metformin inhibits the anti-inflammatory pathway required for transformation and cancer stem cells formation [88].

Further mechanism of anticancer effect of metformin is modulation of microRNAs (miRNAs) expression (mainly tumor suppressor miRNA) through activation and upregulation of the RNAase III endonuclease (DICER). DICER is one of the key enzymes of microRNAs biosynthesis [89]. DICER has a role in formation of miRNAs and in assembly of their machinery to target mRNAs for degradation [90]. Downregulation of DICER is oncogenic and predict poor survival in lung, breast and ovarian cancer [91, 92]. In addition, impairment of metformin effect in vitro was shown in DICER-deficient tumor cells. As shown in **Figure 5**, metformin induced upregulation of DICER leads to expression of many suppressor miRNAs that target mRNA of coding genes for degradation, thus effectively reducing gene products such as oncogenic proteins [93].

6. Mechanisms of action in PCOS

One of the pleiotropic effects of metformin is to reduce insulin resistance (IR) and secondary hyperinsulinemia in diabetes mellitus and several clinical conditions associated with hyperinsulinemia. Hyperinsulinemia is linked with the pathogenesis of polycystic ovary syndrome (PCOS), a condition of primary ovulatory disfunction associated with metabolic disturbances. PCOS is the endocrine disorder characterized by hyperandrogenism, anovulation and infertility. Obesity further exaggerates IR in obese PCOS women. Importantly, IR in PCOs women is tissue selective, which means persistence sensitivity to insulin actions on steroidogenesis in ovary and adrenal gland, in face of resistance in skeletal muscle, adipose tissue and liver to metabolic actions of insulin. Paradoxically, in PCOS women, some tissues manifest IR, while steroid-producing tissues remain insulin sensitive [94].

Mechanisms of insulin action contributing to hyperandrogenism in PCOS are various. Insulin can enhance the amplitude of luteinizing hormone (LT) pulses to increase androgen production in theca cells [95] (similarly insulin increases thecal androgen response to LH through direct binding to insulin like growth factor − 1(IGF-1) receptors in theca cells). Also, insulin may stimulate the activity of ovarian cytochrome CYP17 (P450c17) and 17β-hydroxysteroid dehydrogenase (17βHSD) to promote androgen steroidogenesis [96]. In addition, insulin can decease the hepatic synthesis of steroid hormone binding globin (SHBG), which allows more free androgen and estrogen to be available. Finally, insulin inhibits the hepatic production of IGF binding protein-1 (IGFBP-1), which increases IGF-1 in circulation and allows greater local action [97].

Furthermore, increase androgen levels may be linked to decrease adiponectin secretion by adipocyte in PCOS women, thereby further increasing insulin resistance and subsequently insulin levels [98]. In addition, insulin may affect female subcutaneous adipose tissue and generate androgen from adipocytes by increasing the activity of aldo-keto reductase IC3 (AKRIC3) [99].

Metformin can ameliorate all the above-mentioned actions of insulin in PCOS. Treatment with metformin is useful in reduction of both hyperinsulinemia and circulating androgens and also restores ovarian function with the benefits of increase ovulation, reduce serum androgen levels and improve menstrual cyclicity.

Metformin acts directly on ovarian theca cells and suppresses androgen production by inhibition the enzymatic activity of P450c17 and 17βHSD [100] or indirectly via reduction of hyperinsulinemia and IR by multiple mechanisms. It has been shown that the metabolic actions of metformin on cells include increase in tissue responsiveness to insulin action, insulin receptor numbers in skeletal muscle and adipose tissue, tyrosine kinase activity and glucose uptake. Also, metformin decreases intestinal glucose absorption, plasma glucagon levels, gluconeogenesis and glycogenolysis in the liver. Most of these actions have been mediated through activation of AMPK cascade, which result in indirect reduction of hyperinsulinemia and IR the main pathogenic component in PCOS [101].

By means of anti-inflammatory/antioxidant mechanisms contributing to PCOS, metformin inhibits NF-kB, whose activation triggers IR and inflammation in PCOS [102]. Moreover, metformin increases the activity of the antioxidant enzymes such as catalase and CuZn superoxide dismutase, thereby, it scavenges the reactive oxygen species such as hydrogen peroxide (H_2O_2), superoxide ($O_2.$) and hydroxyl ($OH.$) radicals, where metformin also directly reacts with the latter one [103]. More other related mechanisms of metformin in PCOS are still unclear and elusive.

7. Conclusion

Based on its multiple mechanisms of action and interference with signaling pathways, metformin represents as a promising potential drug for treating various medical conditions. Furthermore, the beneficial effects arising from these mechanisms can be demonstrated and clarified by substantial basic experiments and clinical trials.

Author details

Samira Abdulla Mahmood
Department of Pharmacology and Toxicology, Faculty of Pharmacy,
Aden University, Aden, Republic of Yemen

Address all correspondence to: samabdulla@yahoo.com

IntechOpen

References

[1] Owen MR, Doran E, Halestrap AP. Evidence that metformin exerts its anti-diabetic effects through inhibition of complex 1 of the mitochondrial respiratory chain. Biochem J 2000; 348:607-614.

[2] Duca FA, Côté CD, Rasmussen BA, Zadeh-Tahmasebi M, Rutter GA, Filippi BM, et al. Metformin activates a duodenal AMPK-dependent pathway to lower hepatic glucose production in rats. Nat. Med. 2015; 21:506-511. doi: 10.1038/nm.3787.

[3] Zhou G, Myers R, Li Y, Chen Y, Shen X, Fenyk-Melody J, et al. Role of AMP-activated protein kinase in mechanism of metformin action. J. Clin. Invest. 2001;108: 1167-1174. doi: 10.1172/JCI13505.

[4] Kalender A, Selvaraj A, Kim SY, Gulati P, Brûlé S, Viollet B, et al. Metformin, independent of AMPK, inhibits mTORC1 in a rag GTPasedependent manner. Cell Metab. 2010; 11: 390-401. doi: 10.1016/j.cmet.2010.03.014.

[5] Al-Oanzi ZH, Fountana S, Moonira T, Tudhope SJ, Petrie JL, Alshawi A, Patman J, Arden C, Reeves HL, Agius L. Opposite effects of a glucokinase activator and metformin on glucose-regulated gene expression in hepatocytes. Diabetes Obesity and Metabolism 2017; doi: http://dx.doi.org/10.1111/dom.12910.

[6] Madiraju AK, Erion DM, Rahimi Y, Zhang XM, Braddock DT, Albright RA, et al. Metformin suppresses gluconeogenesis by inhibiting mitochondrial glycerophosphate dehydrogenase. Nature 2014; 510: 542-546. doi: 10.1038/nature13270

[7] Saitoh R, Sugano K, Takata N, Tachibana T, Higashida A, Nabuchi Y and Aso Y. Correction of permeability with pore radius of tight junctions in Caco-2 monolayers improves the prediction of the dose fraction of hydrophilic drugs absorbed by humans. Pharm Res 2004; 21:749-755.

[8] Shu Y , Sheardown SA , Brown C , Owen RP , Zhang S , Castro RA , Ianculescu AG , Yue L , Lo JC , Burchard EG , Brett CM , Giacomini KM . Effect of genetic variation in the organic cation transporter 1 (OCT1) on metformin action . J Clin Invest 2007; 117 : 1422 – 1431.

[9] Koepsell H, Endou H. The SLC22 drug transporter family. Pflugers Arch 2004; 447:666-676

[10] El-Mir MY, Nogueira V, Fontaine E, Averet N, Rigoulet M, Leverve X. Dimethylbiguanide inhibits cell respiration via an indirect effect targeted on the respiratory chain complex I. J Biol Chem 2000; 275:223-228.

[11] Hawley SA, Ross FA, Chevtzoff C, Green KA, Evans A, Fogarty S, et al. Use of cells expressing gamma subunit variants to identify diverse mechanisms of AMPK activation. Cell Metab 2010; 11:554-565.

[12] LaMoia TE, Shulman GI. Cellular and Molecular Mechanisms of Metformin Action. Endocrine Reviews, 2021; 42(1):77-96. doi:10.1210/endrev/bnaa023

[13] Woods A, Johnstone SR, Dickerson K, et al. LKB1 is the upstream kinase in the AMP-activated protein kinase cascade. Curr Biol. 2003;13(22): 2004-2008.

[14] Meng S, Cao J, He Q, Xiong L, Chang E, Radovick S, et al. Metformin activates AMP-activated protein kinase by promoting formation of the abg heterotrimeric complex. J. Biol. Chem.

2015; 290: 3793-3802. doi: 10.1074/jbc.
M114.604421.

[15] Garcia D and Shaw RJ. AMPK:
Mechanisms of Cellular Energy Sensing
and Restoration of Metabolic Balance.
Mol Cell 2017; 66:789-800.

[16] Scott JW, Hawley SA, Green KA, et
al. CBS domains form energy-sensing
modules whose binding of adenosine
ligands is disrupted by disease
mutations. J Clin Invest.
2004;113(2):274-284.

[17] Rosso P, Fioramonti M, Fracassi A,
Marangoni M, Taglietti V, Siteni S,
Segatto M. AMPK in the central nervous
system: physiological roles and
pathological implications. Research and
Report in Biology 2017;7:1-13.

[18] Hardie DG, Ross FA and Hawley SA.
AMPK: A nutrient and energy sensor
that maintains energy homeostasis. Nat
Rev Mol Cell Biol 2012;13: 251-262.

[19] Mihaylova MM and Shaw RJ. The
AMPK signaling pathway coordinates
cell growth, autophagy and metabolism.
Nat Cell Biol 2011;13: 1016-1023.

[20] Wang DS, Jonker JW, Kato Y,
Kusuhara H, Schinkel AH, Sugiyama Y.
Involvement of organic cation
transporter 1 in hepatic and intestinal
distribution of metformin. J Pharmacol
Exp Ther 2002;302:510-515.

[21] Rena G, Hardie DG, Pearson ER.
The mechanisms of action of
metformin. Diabetologia 2017; 60:1577-
1585. doi 10.1007/s00125-017-4342-z.

[22] Pryor HJ, Smyth JE, Quinlan PT,
Halestrap AP. Evidence that the flux
control coefficient of the respiratory
chain is high during gluconeogenesis
from lactate in hepatocytes from starved
rats. Implications for the hormonal
control of gluconeogenesis and action of
hypoglycemic agents. Biochem J
1987;247:449-457.

[23] Foretz M, Hebrard S, Leclerc J,
Zarrinpashneh E, Soty M, Mithieux G,
et al. Metformin inhibits hepatic
gluconeogenesis in mice independently
of the LKB1/AMPK pathway via a
decrease in hepatic energy state. JClin
Invest 2010;120:2355-2369.

[24] Bridges HR, Jones AJ, Pollak MN,
Hirst J. Effects of metformin and other
biguanides on oxidative
phosphorylation in mitochondria.
Biochem J 2014;462:475-487.

[25] Kahn BB, Alquier T, Carling D,
Hardie DG. AMP-activated protein
kinase: Ancient energy gauge provides
clues to modern understanding of
metabolism Cell Metab 2005; 1(1):15-25.

[26] Ross FA, MacKintosh C, Hardie DG.
AMP-activated protein kinase: a cellular
energy sensor that comes in 12 flavours.
FEBS J 2016;283:2987-3001.

[27] Zhou G, Myers R, Li Y, Chen Y,
Shen X, Fenyk-Melody J, et al. Role of
AMP-activated protein kinase in
mechanism of metformin action. J Clin
Invest 2001;108:1167-1174.

[28] Zhang CS, Li M, Ma T, Zong Y,
Cui J, Feng JE, et al. Metformin activates
AMPK through the lysosomal pathway.
Cell Metab 2016;24:521-522

[29] Valencia WM, Palacio A, Tamariz L,
Florez H. (2017) Metformin and ageing:
improving ageing outcomes beyond
glycaemic control. Diabetologia 2017.
doi:10.1007/s00125-017-4349-5.

[30] Patel K, Foretz M, Marion A,
Campbell DG, Gourlay R, Boudaba N, et
al. The LKB1-salt-inducible kinase
pathway functions as a key
gluconeogenic suppressor in the liver.
Nat Commun 2014; 5:4535.

[31] Viollet B, Guigas B, Garcia NS,
Leclerc J, Foretz M, Andreelli F,et al.
Cellular and molecular mechanisms of

metformin: an overview. Clinical Science, Portland Press, 2012; 122(6): 253-270.

[32] Fullerton MD, Galic S, Marcinko K, Sikkema S, Pulinikunnil T, Chen ZP, et al. Single phosphorylation sites in ACC1 and ACC2 regulate lipid homeostasis and the insulin-sensitizing effects of metformin. Nat Med 2013;19:1649-1654.

[33] Foretz M, Ancellin N, Andreelli F, Saintillan Y, Grondin P, Kahn A, *et al.* Short-term overexpression of a constitutively active form of AMP-activated protein kinase in the liver leads to mild hypoglycemia and fatty liver. Diabetes 2005; 54: 1331-1339.

[34] Miller RA , Birnbaum MJ . An energetic tale of AMPK-independent effects of metformin . J Clin Invest. 2010;120: 2267 – 2270.

[35] Miller RA, Chu Q, Xie J, Foretz M, Viollet B, Birnbaum MJ. Biguanides suppress hepatic glucagon signaling by decreasing production of cyclic AMP. Nature 2013;494:256-260.

[36] Jitrapakdee S, St Maurice M, Rayment I, Cleland WW, Wallace JC, Attwood PV. Structure, mechanism and regulation of pyruvate carboxylase. Biochem J. 2008;413(3):369-387.

[37] Perry RJ, Camporez JG, Kursawe R, Titchenell PM, Zhang D, Perry CJ, et al. Hepatic acetyl CoA links adipose tissue inflammation to hepatic insulin resistance and type 2 diabetes. Cell. 2015;160(4):745-758.

[38] Neeland IJ, Hughes C, Ayers CR, Malloy CR, Jin ES. Effects of visceral adiposity on glycerol pathways in gluconeogenesis. Metabolism. 2017;67:80-89.

[39] Cusi K, Consoli A, DeFronzo RA. Metabolic effects of metformin on glucose and lactate metabolism in noninsulin-dependent diabetes mellitus.

J Clin Endocrinol Metab 1996; 81: 4059-4067.

[40] Jager S, Handschin C, St Pierre J, Spiegelman BM. AMP-activated protein kinase (AMPK) action in skeletal muscle via direct phosphorylation of PGC-1 α. PNAS 2007; 104(29):12017: 12022.

[41] Beg M, Abdullah N, Thowfeik FS, Altorki NK, McGraw TE. Distinct Akt phosphorylation states are required for insulin regulated Glut4 and Glut1-mediated glucose uptake. eLife. 2017;6:1-22. doi: 10.7554/eLife.26896.

[42] Wang Z, Wang Y, Han Y, Yin Q, Hu S, Zhao T, et al. Akt is a critical node of acute myocardial insulin resistance and cardiac dysfunction after cardiopulmonary bypass. Life Sciences. 2019;234:116734. doi: 10.1016/j.lfs.2019.116734.

[43] Garabadu D, Krishnamurthy S. Metformin attenuates hepatic insulin resistance in type-2 diabetic rats through PI3K/Akt/GLUT-4 signalling independent to bicuculline-sensitive GABAA receptor stimulation. Pharmaceutical Biology. 2017;55:722-728. doi: 10.1080/13880209.2016.1268635.

[44] Ikeda T, Iwata K, Murakami H. Inhibitory effect of metformin on intestinal glucose absorption in the perfused rat intestine. Biochem Pharmacol 2000; 59: 887-890.

[45] Sakar Y, Meddah B, Faouzi MA, Cherrah Y, Bado A, Ducroc R. Metformin-induced regulation of the intestinal D-glucose. Physiol Pharmacol 2010;61(3):301-307.

[46] McCreight LJ, Bailey CJ, Pearson ER. Metformin and the gastrointestinal tract Diabetologia 2016; 59:426-435. doi 10.1007/s00125-015-3844-9.

[47] Lalau JD, Lacroix C, Compagnon P, de Cagny P, Rigaud JP, Bleichner G, et al.

Role of metformin accumulation in metformin-associated lactic acidosis. Diabetes Care 1995;18:779-784.

[48] Wu T, Thazhath SS, Bound MJ, Jones KL, Horowitz M, Rayner CK. Mechanism of increase in plasma intact GLP-1 by metformin in type 2 diabetes: stimulation of GLP-1 secretion or reduction in plasma DPP-4 activity? Diabetes Res Clin Pract 2014;106:e3–e6.

[49] Cuthbertson J, Patterson S, O'Harte FP, Bell PM. Investigation of the effect of oral metformin on dipeptidylpeptidase-4 (DPP-4) activity in type 2 diabetes. Diabet Med 2009;26:649-654.

[50] Lien F, Berthier A, Bouchaert E, Gheeraert C, Alexandre J, Porez G, et al. Metformin interferes with bile acid homeostasis through AMPK–FXR crosstalk. J Clin Invest 2014;124:1037-1051

[51] Thomas C, Gioiello A, Noriega L, Strehle A, Oury J, Rizzo G, et al. TGR5-mediated bile acid sensing controls glucose homeostasis. Cell Metab 2009;10:167-177

[52] Carter D, Howlett HC, Wiernsperger NF, Bailey CJ. Differential effects of metformin on bile salt absorption from the jejunum and ileum. Diabetes Obes Metab 2003;5:120-125.

[53] Scarpello JH, Hodgson E, Howlett HC. Effect of metformin on bile salt circulation and intestinal motility in type 2 diabetes mellitus. Diabet Med 1998;15:651-656.

[54] Tilg H, Moschen AR. Microbiota and diabetes: an evolving relationship. Gut 2014;63:1513-1521

[55] Yerevanian A and Soukas AA. Metformin: Mechanisms in Human Obesity and Weight Loss Curr Obes Rep. 2019; 8(2): 156-164. doi:10.1007/s13679-019-00335-3.

[56] Morrison DJ and Preston T, Formation of short chain fatty acids by the gut microbiota and their impact on human metabolism. Gut Microbes, 2016;7(3):189-200.

[57] Everard A, Belzer C, Geurts L, Ouwerkerk JP, Druart C, Bindels LB, et al . Cross-talk between Akkermansia muciniphila and intestinal epithelium controls dietinduced obesity. Proc Natl Acad Sci U S A 2013; 110:9066-9071

[58] Sena CM, Matafome P, Louro T, Nunes E, Fernandes R, Seica RM. Metformin restores endothelial function in aorta of diabetic rats. Br J Pharmacol 2011;163: 424-437.

[59] Li SN, Wang X, Zeng QT, Feng YB, Cheng X, Mao XB, et al. Metformin inhibits nuclear factor kappaB activation and decreases serum high-sensitivity C-reactive protein level in experimental atherogenesis of rabbits. Heart Vessels 2009; 24: 446-453.

[60] Hattori Y, Suzuki K, Hattori S, Kasai K. Metformin inhibits cytokine-induced nuclear factor κB activation via AMP-activated protein kinase activation in vascular endothelial cells. Hypertension. 2006;47:1183-1188.

[61] Wang C, Liu C, Gao K, Zhao H, Zhou Z, Shen Z, et al. Metformin preconditioning provide neuroprotection through enhancement of autophagy and suppression of inflammation and apoptosis after spinal cord injury. Biochem Biophys Res Commun. 2016;477:534-540. doi: 10.1016/j.bbrc.2016.05.148.

[62] Chakraborty A, Chowdhury S, Bhattacharyya M. Effect of metformin on oxidative stress, nitrosative stress and inflammatory biomarkers in type 2 diabetes patients. Diabetes Res Clin Pract. 2011;93(1):56-62. doi: 10.1016/j.diabres.2010.11.030.

[63] Vasamsetti SB, Karnewar S, Kanugula AK, Thatipalli AR, Kumar JM,

Kotamraju S. Metformin inhibits monocyte-to-macrophage differentiation via AMPK-mediated inhibition of STAT3 activation: potential role in atherosclerosis. Diabetes. 2015; 64:2028-2041. doi: 10.2337/db14-122.

[64] Hyun B, Shin S, Lee A, Lee S, Song Y, Ha NJ, et al. Metformin down-regulates TNFalpha secretion *via* suppression of scavenger receptors in macrophages. Immune Netw 2013; 13: 123-132.

[65] Koh SJ, Kim JM, Kim IK, Ko SH, Kim JS. Anti-inflammatory mechanism of metformin and its effects in intestinal inflammation and colitis-associated colon cancer. J Gastroenterol Hepatol. 2014;29:502-510.

[66] Esteves CL, Kelly V, Breton A, Taylor AI, West CC, Donadeu FX, et al. Proinflammatory cytokine induction of 11beta-hydroxysteroid dehydrogenase type 1 (11beta- HSD1) in human adipocytes is mediated by MEK, C/EBPbeta, and NF-kappaB/RelA. J Clin Endocrinol Metab 2014; 99: E160-E168.

[67] Xiao Z, Wu W, Poltoratsky V. Metformin Suppressed CXCL8 Expression and Cell Migration in HEK293/TLR4 Cell Line. Mediators Inflamm. 2017; 2017:6589423. doi: 10.1155/2017/6589423.

[68] Dehkordi AH, Abbaszadeh A, Mir S, Hasanvand A. Metformin and its anti-inflammatory and anti-oxidative effects; new concepts. J Renal Inj Prev. 2019;8(1):54-61. doi: 10.15171/jrip.2019.11.

[69] Hattori Y, Hattori K, Hayashi T. Pleiotropic Benefits of Metformin: Macrophage Targeting Its Anti-inflammatory Mechanisms Diabetes 2015;64:1907-1909 doi: 10.2337/db15-0090.

[70] Beisswenger P, Ruggiero-Lopez D. Metformin inhibition of glycation processes. Diabetes Metab 2003; 29: 6S95-6103.

[71] Ramasamy R, Yan SF, Schmidt AM. The diverse ligand repertoire of the receptor for advanced glycation endproducts and pathways to the complications of diabetes. Vascul Pharmacol 2012; 57: 160-167.

[72] Basta G. Receptor for advanced glycation endproducts and atherosclerosis: From basic mechanisms to clinical implications. Atherosclerosis 2008; 196: 9-21.

[73] Saisho Y. Metformin and Inflammation: Its Potential Beyond Glucose-lowering Effect Endocrine, Metabolic & Immune Disorders, Drug Targets, 2015;15:1-10.

[74] Gamad N, Malik S, Suchal K, Vasisht S, Tomar A, Arava S, et al. Metformin alleviates bleomycin-induced pulmonary fibrosis in rats: Pharmacological effects and molecular mechanisms. Biomed Pharmacother. 2018;97:1544-1553.

[75] Franciosi, M., Lucisano, G., Lapice, E., Strippoli, G. F., Pellegrini, F., Nicolucci, A. Metformin therapy and risk of cancer in patients with type 2 diabetes: systematic review. PLoS One 2013;8:e71583. doi: 10.1371/journal.pone.0071583

[76] Zhang, P., Li, H., Tan, X., Chen, L., and Wang, S. Association of metformin use with cancer incidence and mortality: a meta-analysis. Cancer Epidemiol. 2013;37, 207-218. doi: 10.1016/j.canep.2012.12.009.

[77] Hou, G., Zhang, S., Zhang, X., Wang, P., Hao, X., and Zhang, J. Clinical pathological characteristics and prognostic analysis of 1,013 breast cancer patients with diabetes. Breast Cancer Res. Treat. 2013;137, 807-816. doi: 10.1007/s10549-012-2404-y.

[78] Yi, Y., Gao, L., Wu, M., Ao, J., Zhang, C., Wang, X., et al. (2017). Metformin sensitizes leukemia cells to vincristine via activation of AMP-activated protein kinase. J. Cancer 2017;8, 2636-2642. doi: 10.7150/jca.19873.

[79] Candido, S., Abrams, S. L., Steelman, L., Lertpiriyapong, K., Martelli, A. M., Cocco, L., et al. Metformin influences drug sensitivity in pancreatic cancer cells. Adv Biol Regul. 2018;68:13-30. doi: 10.1016/j.jbior.2018.02.002.

[80] Mu N, Xu T, Gao M, Dong M, Therapeutic effect of metformin in the treatment of endometrial cancer (Review) Oncology Letters 2020 ;20:156.doi: 10.3892/ol.2020.12017.

[81] Jones, R. G., Plas, D. R., Kubek, S., Buzzai, M., Mu, J., and Xu, Y. AMP activated protein kinase induces a p53-dependent metabolic checkpoint. Mol. Cell 2005;18: 283-293. doi: 10.1016/j.molcel.2005.03.027.

[82] He G, Zhang YW, Lee JH, Zeng SX, Wang YV, Luo Z, Dong XG, Viollet B, Wahl GM, Lua H. AMP-Activated Protein Kinase Induces p53 by Phosphorylating MDMX and Inhibiting Its Activity. Molecular and Cellular Biology 2014;34(2):148-157.

[83] Hilliard S, Aboudehen K, Yao X, El-Dahr SS. Tight regulation of p53 activity by Mdm2 is required for ureteric bud growth and branching. Dev. Biol. 2011;353:354-366.

[84] Saxton, RA and Sabatini DM. mTOR signaling in growth, metabolism, and disease. Cell 2017;168: 960-976. doi: 10.1016/j.cell.2017.02.004.

[85] Rosso P, Fioramonti M, Fracassi A, Marangoni M, Taglietti V, Siteni S, Segatto M. AMPK in the central nervous system: physiological roles and pathological implications. Research and Reports in Biology 2016;7: 1-13.

[86] Inoki K, Zhu T, Guan KL. TSC2 mediates cellular energy response to control cell growth and survival. Cell. 2003;115(5):577-590.

[87] Roncolato F, Lindemann K, Willson ML, Martyn J and Mileshkin L: PI3K/AKT/mTOR inhibitors for advanced or recurrent endometrial cancer. Cochrane Database Syst Rev 2019;10:CD012160.

[88] Hirsch HA, Iliopoulos D, Struhl K. Metformin inhibits the inflammatory response associated with cellular transformation and cancer stem cell growth. PNAS 2013; 110 (3) www.pnas.org/cgi/doi/10.1073/pnas.1221055110.

[89] Bernstein E, Caudy AA, Hammond SM. Hannon GJ. Role for a bidentate ribonuclease in the initiation step of RNA interference. Nature 2001; 409, 363-366.

[90] Kim VN. MicroRNA biogenesis: coordinated cropping and dicing. Nat Rev Mol Cell Biol. 2005; 6:376-385.

[91] Martello G, Rosato A, Ferrari F, Manfrin A, Cordenonsi M, Dupont S, et al. A MicroRNA targeting DICER for metastasis control. Cell 2010;141: 1195-1207.

[92] Merritt WM, Lin YG, Han LY, Kamat AA, Spannuth WA, Schmandt R, et al. DICER, Drosha, and outcomes in patients with ovarian cancer. N. Engl. J. Med. 2008; 359, 2641-2650.

[93] Blandino G, Valerio M, Cioce M, Mori F, Casadei L, Pulito C, Sacconi A et al. Metformin elicits anticancer effects through the sequential modulation of DICER and c-MYC. Nature Communications 2012. doi: 10.1038/ncomms1859.

[94] Geffner ME, Golde DW: Selective insulin action on skin, ovary, and heart in insulin-resistant states. Diabetes Care 1988;11:500-505.

[95] Willis D, Franks S: Insulin action in human granulosa cells from normal and polycystic ovaries is mediated by the insulin receptor and not the type-I insulin-like growth factor receptor. J Clin Endocrinol Metab 1995; 80: 3788-3790.

[96] Adashi EY, Hsueh AJW, Yen SSC: Insulin enhancement of luteinizing hormone and follicle stimulating hormone release by cultured pituitary cells. Endocrinology 1981; 108: 1441-1449.

[97] Le Roith D, McGuinness M, Shemer J, Stannard B, Lanau F, Faria TN, Kato H, Werner H, Adamo M, Roberts Jr CT. Insulin like growth factors. Biology Signals, 1992;1:173-181.

[98] O'Connor A, Phelan N, Tun TK, Boran G, Gibney J, Roche HM: High-molecular-weight adiponectin is selectively reduced in women with polycystic ovary syndrome independent of body mass index and severity of insulin resistance. J Clin Endocrinol Metab 2010; 95: 1378-1385.

[99] O'Reilly M, Gathercole L, Capper F, Arlt W, Tomlinson J: Effect of insulin on AKR1C3 expression in female adipose tissue: in-vivo and in-vitro study of adipose androgen generation in polycystic ovary syndrome. Lancet 2015; 385(suppl 1):S16.

[100] Hirsch A, Hahn D, Kempna P, Hofer G, Nuoffer JM, Mullis PE, et al. Metformin inhibits human androgen production by regulating steroidogenic enzymes HSD3B2 and CYP17A1 and complex I activity of the respiratory chain. Endocrinology. 2012;153: 4354-4366. doi: 10.1210/en.2012-1145.

[101] Dumitrescu R, Mehedintu C, Briceag I, Purcarea VL, Hudita D. Metformin-Clinical Pharmacology in PCOs. Journal of Medicine and Life 2015;8(2):187-192.

[102] Gonzalez F, Rote NS, Minium J, Kirwan JP. Increased activation of nuclear factor kappa B triggers inflammation and insulin resistance in polycystic ovary syndrome. J Clin Endocrinol Metab 2006; 91(4): 1508-1512.

[103] Motta AB. Mechanisms Involved in Metformin Action in the Treatment of Polycystic Ovary Syndrome. Current Pharmaceutical Design, 2009;15: 3074-3077.

Chapter 2

Prevention of Hyperglycemia

Lucy A. Ochola and Eric M. Guantai

Abstract

Hyperglycemia is the elevation of blood glucose concentrations above the normal range. Prolonged uncontrolled hyperglycemia is associated with serious life-threatening complications. Hyperglycemia arises from an imbalance between glucose production and glucose uptake and utilization by peripheral tissues. Disorders that compromise pancreatic function or affect the glucose counter-regulatory hormones cause hyperglycemia. Acute or serious illness or injury may also bring about hyperglycemia, as can many classes of drugs. Metformin lowers blood glucose levels by inhibiting the production of glucose by the liver whilst enhancing uptake of circulating glucose and its utilization in peripheral tissues such as muscle and adipose tissue. Metformin suppresses hepatic gluconeogenesis by inhibiting mitochondrial respiration and causing a reduction of cellular ATP levels. Metformin may also modulate the gut-brain-liver axis, resulting in suppression of hepatic glucose production. Metformin also opposes the hyperglycemic action of glucagon and may ameliorate pancreatic cell dysfunction associated with hyperglycemia. Metformin is therefore recommended for use in the prevention of hyperglycemia, including drug-induced hyperglycemia, in at risk patients. The benefits of metformin in the prevention of hyperglycemia are unmatched despite its contraindications.

Keywords: hyperglycemia, hyperinsulinemia, insulin, metformin, glucose

1. Introduction

Chronic hyperglycemia can lead to complications involving damage to the kidneys, retina, nervous system and cardiovascular system. In this chapter, we discuss the causes of hyperglycemia, including drug-induced hyperglycemia, highlighting the importance and approaches to prevention and management of hyperglycemia. We focus on the role and rationale for the use of metformin for the prevention of hyperglycemia, presenting the evidence that supports its use for this indication.

2. Hyperglycemia

Hyperglycemia, which literally means 'high blood glucose' levels, refers to the elevation of blood glucose concentrations above the normal range. Specifically, it refers to fasting blood glucose levels greater than 7.0 mmol/L (126 mg/dl) or 2-hour postprandial blood glucose levels greater than 11.0 mmol/L (200 mg/dl) [1].

2.1 Symptoms and complications

Mild, transient hyperglycemia is largely asymptomatic. However, prolonged uncontrolled hyperglycemia is associated with various symptoms including the classic hyperglycemic triad of polyuria, polydipsia, and polyphagia, as well as blurred vision, dehydration, weight changes (gain or loss), generalized fatigue, abdominal discomfort, nausea, vomiting and muscle cramps [1, 2]. Complications arise when the hyperglycemia is severe and/or persists over an extended period. Frequent infections, erectile dysfunction and poor wound healing are associated with prolonged hyperglycemia. Chronic hyperglycemia can also lead to many serious life-threatening complications involving damage to the kidneys (nephropathy), retina (retinopathy), nervous system (peripheral neuropathy) and cardiovascular system (myocardial infarction, stroke) [1–5].

2.2 Causes of hyperglycemia

Blood glucose levels reflect the dynamic balance between, on the one hand, dietary glucose absorption and hepatic glucose production and, on the other hand, glucose uptake and utilization by peripheral tissues. Except for dietary glucose absorption, these complex and interrelated processes are under the control of the hormone insulin and, to a lesser extent, other counter-regulatory hormones such as glucagon, catecholamines, cortisol and growth hormone [1, 6]. Hyperglycemia arises from an imbalance in these processes that determine blood glucose levels.

The greatest quantitative determinant for hyperglycemia is dysfunction in pancreatic islet cell activity which affects insulin release from the pancreas in response to. The pathophysiology of hyperglycemia also entails a resulting degree of insulin resistance and impairment in homeostatic glucose regulation. Insulin resistance results in decreased uptake of glucose by insulin-sensitive tissues as well as a consequential increase in endogenous glucose production. This all leads to hyperglycemia [7]. The elevation of blood glucose levels during the fasting state is directly proportional to the increase in hepatic glucose production while that of the postprandial state is connected to insufficient suppression of glucose output plus a defect in the stimulation of insulin hormone on recipient tissues like skeletal muscle [8].

The progression of this imbalance in blood glucose homeostasis over time leads to the development of diabetes, a chronic disease affecting glucose metabolism that occurs due to either insufficient production of insulin by the pancreas, or inadequate response by tissues to insulin [9]. The development of diabetes can be delayed or prevented by targeting the early prevention and/or reversal of hyperglycemia, as well as by inhibiting the development of hyperinsulinemia-induced insulin resistance [10]. This would also delay progression of prediabetic states to diabetes [11].

In addition to diabetes, there are a myriad of other causes of hyperglycemia, i.e., non-diabetic hyperglycemia. Disorders that compromise pancreatic function (pancreatic cancer, cystic fibrosis, chronic pancreatitis, etc.) or affect the glucose counter-regulatory hormones (pheochromocytoma, acromegaly, Cushing syndrome) cause hyperglycemia. Transient hyperglycemia may arise consequent to abnormally high carbohydrates in the diet, dextrose infusion and total parental nutrition. Acute or serious illness or injury may also bring about transient hyperglycemia referred to as stress hyperglycemia or hospital-related hyperglycemia [1, 12].

Medicines may also induce hyperglycemia [1, 6, 13].

2.3 Drug-induced hyperglycemia

Drug-induced hyperglycemia refers to the clinically relevant elevation of blood glucose levels caused by drugs [13]. Whereas drug-induced hyperglycemia is often mild and asymptomatic, severe hyperglycemia may occur particularly in predisposed patients, such as those with pre-existing pancreatic dysfunction or insulin resistance. Drug-induced hyperglycemia can occur in adults and children alike, and certain patient factors are known to increase the risk of drug-induced hyperglycemia, such as obesity, sedentary lifestyle, stress, illness, history of gestational diabetes, or a family history of diabetes [6, 14].

Many classes of drugs have been implicated in causing hyperglycemia via various mechanisms. Some drugs cause hyperglycemia by reducing insulin production/secretion (glucocorticoids, β-receptor antagonists, thiazide diuretics, calcium-channel blockers, phenytoin, pentamidine, calcineurin inhibitors, protease inhibitors), including by direct damage to pancreatic cells (glucocorticoids, pentamidine, statins). Glucocorticoids, β-receptor antagonists and thiazide diuretics also promote hepatic glucose production and reduce insulin sensitivity. Other classes of drugs that reduce peripheral tissue sensitivity to insulin include atypical antipsychotics, antidepressants, oral contraceptives, statins, nucleoside reverse transcriptase inhibitors and protease inhibitors [1, 6, 14–16]. Hyperglycemia is one of the common adverse effects of the anticancer agent L-asparaginase, which inhibits insulin synthesis by depleting available asparagine in pancreatic cells in addition to impairing insulin receptor activity and promoting peripheral tissue resistance to insulin [14]. Monoclonal antibodies such as nivolumab and pembrolizumab may cause severe hyperglycemia by triggering the autoimmune-mediated destruction of pancreatic cells [17, 18]. β2-receptor agonists cause hyperglycemia by promoting hepatic and

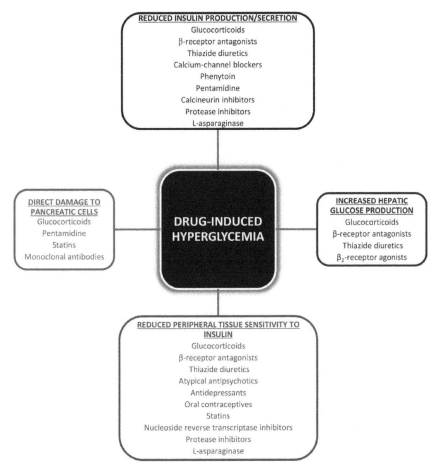

Figure 1.
Mechanisms of drug-induced hyperglycemia and implicated classes of drugs.

muscle glucose production [19]. The various mechanisms of drug-induced hyperglycemia and the classes of drugs implicated are shown in **Figure 1**.

The overall occurrence of drug-induced hyperglycemia is not known and would obviously vary between individual drugs. There is a lack of data on the burden of drug-induced hyperglycemia for specific drugs, and a few studies have attempted to address this gap. For example, the incidence of corticosteroid-related hyperglycemia in patients treated with high dose corticosteroids has been estimated to be in excess 50% [20, 21]. Comparably high prevalence has been reported for clozapine [22]. These and other similar findings strongly suggest that the risk of drug-induced hyperglycemia (alongside the risk of new-onset diabetes) is real.

The onset of drug-induced hyperglycemia varies on the medication administered. At the time of or shortly after initiating corticosteroids, blood glucose levels may be altered, whereas patients on hydrochlorothiazide may not experience altered levels for weeks or longer, depending on the dose given. In regard to second generation antipsychotics (SGAs), a consensus statement developed by the American Diabetes Association (ADA) in conjunction with other medical organizations recommends monitoring fasting blood glucose for 12 weeks after initiation of therapy and annually thereafter in those without diabetes. However, cases involving hyperglycemic crises have been reported within weeks of starting SGAs [23].

3. Prevention and management of hyperglycemia

The common medical occurrence of hyperglycemic states has yet to be given the due attention it deserves, considering the numerous consequences it bears to patients and the healthcare fraternity. The existing reality of numerous patients suffering from hyperglycemia of varied cause provides an overwhelming patient load, unmatched by the number of specialized providers. However, the management of hyperglycemia has continually posed a great challenge mainly from a lack of standardized protocols [24]. Currently, lack of knowledge and consensus on strategies of management play a significant role in its mismanagement.

Insulin resistance and the resulting compensatory hyperinsulinemia is considered to preclude the development of type 2 diabetes. Hyperglycemia prophylaxis is thus highly attractive based on the numerous socio-economic benefits it confers to patients and the healthcare system. Several studies have demonstrated the advantages gained from preventing elevations of blood glucose levels across a divergent patient portfolio. Research has broadly focused on management of hyperglycemia regardless of the cause, which underlies the common pathways involved in the development of hyperglycemia.

3.1 The role of insulin

The primary strategy employed in hyperglycemia management is insulin [25]. Consensus arrived at by ADA and European Association for the Study of Diabetes (EASD) outline the management of hyperglycemia in type 2 diabetes patients. These guidelines have also been adopted in the prevention of hyperglycemia from other causes, including drug-induced hyperglycemia. The guidelines recommend the use of insulin in all hospitalized patients, with discontinuation of oral hypoglycemic medication [26, 27]. Stoppage of the drugs is on the basis that majority of hospitalized patients present with concurrent conditions and/or physiological dysfunctions that tend to contraindicate continued use of these medications if already prescribed. The pharmacokinetics of oral medication, which tend to have a slow onset of action, disallows for rapid dose adjustment to changing patient needs [28].

Therefore, it is recommended that critically ill patients be treated with a continuous insulin infusion while non-critically ill patients are initiated on subcutaneous (SC) insulin. An individualized dose adjustment for insulin is advised across major studies [26, 29]. Resumption of oral diabetic agents (ODA) when transitioning from inpatient to outpatient setting, with careful consideration given to previous insulin dosing, is advised upon successful treatment. A study involving patients without diabetes recommended the administration of intravenous (IV) insulin infusion in patients with serum blood glucose level values of greater than 10 mmol/L, with a target of achieving serum blood glucose levels of 7.8–10 mmol/L in non-critical settings and less than 7.8 mmol/L in an outpatient setting [30].

Despite numerous recommendations, challenges faced by providers during insulin administration cannot be overlooked. The biggest impediment to insulin use in management of drug-induced hyperglycemia in the affected population is the unavoidable side effect of hypoglycemia [31]. Unfortunately, insulin treatment is the most common risk factor for inpatient hypoglycemia. The incidence of hypoglycemia is approximately 30% in elderly patients, in spite of using low dose insulin and oral diabetic agents [28]. This is associated with increased mortality rate and prolonged hospital stays. Hence, constant monitoring of blood glucose levels is necessary.

Dose adjustments using patients' weight is perceived to be safe and effective as long as close monitoring is done. However, this is not always feasible, let alone practical with many patients. So too is the recommendation of individualizing glycemic targets for patients based on clinical status, risk of hypoglycemia and patient comorbidities, no matter the benefit it confers. This is because the number of patients with drug-induced hyperglycemia cannot be matched to the number of specialized health care workers required to meet this need.

Herein lies the difficulty as many patients are unable to achieve the close monitoring desired, let alone manage the expected side effects in a home-based set up. Even in hospitalized patients, lack of protocols for dose adjustment poses a hindrance in adequate control of elevated blood glucose levels. Hypoglycemia presents a consequential effect that should be carefully considered in hyperglycemia management. Any chosen medication, in addition to lifestyle interventions, should ideally be one that is safe, effective, economical and with minimal side effects.

3.2 The role of oral antidiabetic medications

Non-insulin medications provide a practical alternative to achieving glycemic control. These agents may also confer a non-glycemic benefit whilst regulating the fluctuations in blood glucose levels. Alternatives among non-insulin medication include metformin, sulphonylureas, glinides, thiazolidinediones, glucagon-like peptide-1 (GLP-1) receptor agonists, and sodium–glucose cotransporter2 (SGLT2) inhibitors.

However, the side effects of each of these agents must also be considered. For example, SGLT2 inhibitors reduce blood glucose levels by preventing proximal tubular reabsorption in the kidney. This has been shown to effectively reduce glycated hemoglobin A1c (HbA1c) levels by 0.6–1.0%. They are also associated with a low risk of hypoglycemia. However, the dehydration side effects make these agents contraindicated in renal dysfunction. They also bear an increased risk of urinary and genital tract infections and are related with the development of diabetic keto-acidosis among diabetic patients [32]. Such a profile tends to limit the use of these agents. Metformin use is contraindicated in the presence of any possible indication for iodinated contrast media and in renal insufficiency while thiazolidinediones are associated with fluid retention. On the other hand, sulfonylureas and glinides result in hypoglycemia in most patients while GLP-1 receptor antagonists can cause nausea and hence need to be withheld in critical patients. In spite of the many side effects of oral diabetic agents and the recommendation of using insulin as first line, recent studies have leaned towards the adoption of the oral diabetic agents. The drug most endorsed based on clinical evidence has been metformin [33].

4. Metformin for the prevention of hyperglycemia

4.1 Introduction and rationale

The pathophysiology of hyperglycemia entails a degree of insulin resistance and results in decreased uptake of glucose by insulin-sensitive tissues as well as a consequential increase in endogenous glucose production [7]. Dysfunction in the activity of pancreatic islet cells affects insulin release in response to rising blood glucose levels. Targeting the prevention and/or reversal of dysglycemia and insulin resistance is the principal behind preventing the development of hyperglycemia [11]. Any agent used in prevention of hyperglycemia must therefore target these pathways, thereby partially or completely eliminating its development.

Metformin can rightfully be considered for hyperglycemia prevention and treatment in cases of insulin resistance. Metformin is a first-line agent in treatment of type 2 diabetes mellitus. Recent studies have shown it confers a greater benefit to patients than the other oral diabetic agents, which has led to its recommendation for use in the prevention of hyperglycemia and prediabetes in at risk patients [34–36].

4.2 Mechanisms of action/pharmacodynamics

Metformin prevents hyperglycemia by hastening the clearance of glucose [37, 38]. It causes a reduction in hyperglycemia and hyperinsulinemia [39]. This facilitates a consequent decline in high insulin and high blood glucose levels, with no effect on insulin secretion. The primary mechanism involved in lowering blood glucose levels is through improving hepatic and peripheral tissue sensitivity to insulin [40]. It inhibits the production of glucose by the liver whilst enhancing uptake of circulating glucose and its utilization in peripheral tissues such as muscle and adipose tissue.

Hepatic gluconeogenesis is an energy-demanding process in which synthesis of one molecule of glucose from lactate or pyruvate requires four molecules of ATP and two molecules of GTP. Metformin suppresses hepatic gluconeogenesis by causing a reduction of cellular ATP levels [41]. Molecularly, metformin appears to inhibit mitochondrial respiration. The resulting shift in cellular energy balance increases the activity of AMP-activated protein kinase (AMPK), which promotes the action of insulin and reduces hepatic gluconeogenesis [42]. AMPK acts as a cell energy sensor: it plays a role in energy balance at the cellular and body level by adapting to changes in the concentration of AMP/ADP relative to ATP [43]. Upon activation by a decrease in cellular energy levels, AMPK initiates a change from anabolic to catabolic pathways that consume ATP. This stimulates the uptake and use of glucose and oxidation of fatty acids, in addition to the suppression of hepatic glucose production. Metformin's' inhibition of the mitochondrial complex is the basis of its effect as observed through the change in the ratios of AMP/ATP or ADP/ATP after its administration [44]. Multiple studies have demostrated that one of the mechanisms of action of metformin is the disruption of mitochondrial complex I [45, 46].

Metformin may also modulate the gut-brain-liver axis through the activation of a duodenal AMPK-dependent pathway, as has been demonstrated in rats. This effect involves activation of protein kinase A (Pka) by GLP-1 in duodenal enterocytes, and results in suppression of hepatic glucose production [47]. It has been shown that glucocorticoid therapy leads to changes in the activation of AMPK in Cushing's syndrome patients and in vitro in human adipocytes, effects that were reversed with metformin in human adipocytes. These indicate the likelihood of converse effects of steroids and metformin in the AMPK signaling pathway, as well as the overriding of steroid effects by metformin [44, 48]. Supporting studies demonstrate that steroid-related increase in glucose levels can be prevented with an AMPK activator [49].

Another postulated mechanism of action for metformin is by causing an increase in circulating cyclic adenosine monophosphate (cAMP) which in turn opposes the hyperglycemic action of glucagon [42, 50]. Metformin has also been postulated to increase the concentration of Glucagon-like peptide-1 (GLP-1) by enhancing site production as well as subsequently decreasing its degradation in circulation and specific tissues via inactivation of the enzyme dipeptide peptidase-4 (DPP-4). Additionally, metformin may induce up regulation of GLP-1receptors on beta cell surfaces of the pancreas. This can aid in ameliorating the beta cell dysfunction associated with hyperglycemia via the enhancement of the role of GLP-1 on glucose dependent release of insulin [11].

4.3 Metformin prevents hyperglycemia and hyperinsulinemia

Metformin can rightfully be considered for hyperglycemia prevention and treatment in cases of insulin resistance. Metformin has been identified as a first line agent in treatment of type 2 diabetes mellitus. Recent studies have shown that it confers a greater benefit to patients than the other oral diabetic agents, which has led to its recommendation for use in the prevention of prediabetes in at risk patients [34, 35, 51]. Presently though, only a few nations have formally adopted this proposal such as Poland, Philippines and Turkey but many may adopt it in the near future based on the emerging evidence [11]. Metformin overrides most of the factors that contribute to poor glycemic management like inaccessibility to medicine and fear of developing hypoglycemia. This improves patient perception on its use regardless of the minimal side effects. In addition, it has been demonstrated to confer long term benefit to those who use it prophylactically. A study that followed up patients from a diabetes prevention program after 15 years found that the metformin treatment arm had a 17% lower incidence for developing type 2 diabetes than the placebo arm. This was determined using the HbA1c parameter, in which 36% of the patients had a risk reduction for diabetes development [34].

In a prospective observational study in persons with normal glucose tolerance and hyperinsulinemia, a dose of 2.55 ± 0.2 g/day of metformin restored physiological insulin secretion by decreasing fasting and post-glucose load hyperinsulinemia in the oral glucose tolerance test (OGTT). Over the observation period, the effect of metformin on the reduction of hyperinsulinemia increased over time, peaking after 1 year of treatment. The ability to lower fasting blood glucose levels also improved with time. Fasting blood glucose levels reached normoglycemic range at 3 months and remained so until the end of the 1 year observation period, with no development of hypoglycemia [39]. A substantial decrease in hyperinsulinemia from high blood glucose levels has also been reported in metformin-treated patients based on an increase in the uptake of glucose [52]. The enhancement of insulin action reduces the load on the beta cells in insulin secretion thus can aid in ameliorating the beta cell dysfunction to an extent; this confers an advantage to patients predisposed to developing hyperglycemia.

In addition, a randomized controlled study showed that there was no significant difference in blood glucose levels between critically ill patients receiving 1000 mg of metformin daily versus a similar spectrum of patients receiving 50 International Units (IU) of regular insulin. Furthermore, metformin-treated patients had blood glucose levels subside to near-normal range [40]. The targeted desired blood glucose levels were achieved with metformin after three days while insulin failed to do the same.

4.4 Metformin for drug-induced hyperglycemia

In acute lymphoblastic leukemia patients with drug-induce hyperglycemia, metformin monotherapy controlled blood glucose in 12 out of 17 patients, without the need for insulin using a median dose of 1000 mg/day for a median of 6 days. Blood glucose levels never exceeded 11.1 mmol/L in 8 of the 12 patients. The one patient who developed hyperglycemia during relapse re-induction for leukemia treatment was effectively controlled using metformin alone [53]. Three of the patients given insulin therapy due to high blood glucose levels were eventually weaned off insulin to metformin alone. Additionally, in a controlled trial consisting of non-diabetic patients on glucocorticoids, metformin prevented an increase of 2-hour glucose AUC with, signifying glucose tolerance preservation. No changes in baseline and after 4 weeks metformin treatment was seen with the 2-hour glucose AUC whereas this parameter increased in the placebo group [54].

Similarly, the effect of metformin on prednisone-induced hyperglycemia (PIH) was observed on fasting and 2-hour post prandial glucose levels in hematological cancer patients. The fasting blood glucose readings indicated a proportion of prednisone-induced hyperglycemia of 72.7% and 14.3% in the control and treatment groups respectively. The proportion was slightly lower while using the 2-hour post prandial glucose, in which 54.5% of participants in the control group developed prednisone-induced hyperglycemia while none developed prednisone-induced hyperglycemia in the treatment group. Patients in the control group had 16 (95% CI 1.3–194.6) times the odds of developing prednisone-induced hyperglycemia compared to patients in the treatment group. Double daily dosing (1700 mg twice daily) was more effective in preventing prednisone-induced hyperglycemia [21]. This is supported by other studies that show that that a daily dose of metformin 1500 mg contributes to 80–85% glucose lowering effects [55].

4.5 Metformin for hyperglycemia: risks and benefits

The limitations attached to the full exploitation of metformin use include its relative contraindications in many hospitalized patients who present with comorbidities like renal insufficiency or unstable hemodynamic status. Metformin is contraindicated if serum creatinine is ≥133 mmol/L in men or ≥ 124 mmol/L in women. Emerging evidence shows that the established cut-off points for renal safety may be overly restrictive [56]. It has been argued that there is a need to relax these cut-offs and policies to allow use of this drug to patients with stable chronic kidney disease characterized by mild–moderate renal insufficiency [57–59].

The associated risk of lactic acidosis tends to deter the use of metformin in majority of the comorbid patients on drugs that predispose to the development of hyperglycemia. However, the studies that made such recommendations used a small percentage of the patient population, thus limiting the extrapolation of these recommendations to the greater public [60]. Fortunately, the incidence of metformin-induced lactic acidosis is rare and can be significantly reduced in at-risk patients by observing the necessary precautions [27, 56]. Other factors may also play a greater role in in being predictors of acidosis, such as dehydration, severe heart and renal failure. Thus, its benefits for use outweigh the potential risk of lactic acidosis.

Supporting evidence on avoidance of metformin use in certain cases is poor and inconsistent such as in patients undergoing radio-contrast imaging which theoretically predisposes patients to media-induced nephropathy, increasing the risk of lactic acidosis [56].

The benefits of metformin in the prevention of hyperglycemia are unmatched despite its list of contraindications. This has facilitated its expanded use based on its well-founded glycemic effects as well as numerous benefits conferred such as the beneficial effect on reduction of development of cardiovascular risk factors [61]. It confers good glycemic management that yields a substantial and enduring decrease in the onset and progression of micro vascular complications [60].

Moreover, large based clinical trials and systematic reviews have shown its beneficial effect of enhancing weight loss, even the weight loss associated with medicaments like antipsychotic agents [62, 63].

5. Conclusions

In summary, the suppression of glucose production by metformin's direct effect plus the enhancement of hepatic insulin signaling will curb the development of drug-induced hyperglycemia. Metformin has been shown to reduce the incidence of hyperglycemia-related complications such as diabetes and risk factors for cardiovascular disease in patients with impaired glucose tolerance and fasting blood sugar [11, 64, 65]. This has led to its endorsement of use in patients with high risk of developing the aforementioned conditions [36].

Author details

Lucy A. Ochola[1*] and Eric M. Guantai[2]

1 Machakos Level 5 Hospital, Machakos, Kenya

2 School of Pharmacy, University of Nairobi, Nairobi, Kenya

*Address all correspondence to: lucyochola@gmail.com

IntechOpen

References

[1] Mouri Mi, Badireddy M. Hyperglycemia. In: StatPearls [Internet]. Treasure Island (FL): StatPearls Publishing; 2021 [cited 2021 Jun 17]. Available from: http://www.ncbi.nlm.nih.gov/books/NBK430900/

[2] Utiger RD. Hyperglycemia [Internet]. Encyclopedia Britannica. [cited 2021 Jun 18]. Available from: https://www.britannica.com/science/hyperglycemia

[3] Chao JH, Hirsch IB. Initial Management of Severe Hyperglycemia in Type 2 Diabetes. In: Feingold KR, Anawalt B, Boyce A, Chrousos G, de Herder WW, Dhatariya K, et al., editors. South Dartmouth (MA); 2000.

[4] Cole JB, Florez JC. Genetics of diabetes mellitus and diabetes complications. Nat Rev Nephrol. 2020 Jul;16(7):377-90.

[5] Kautzky-Willer A, Harreiter J, Pacini G. Sex and Gender Differences in Risk, Pathophysiology and Complications of Type 2 Diabetes Mellitus. Endocr Rev. 2016 Jun;37(3):278-316.

[6] Fathallah N, Slim R, Larif S, Hmouda H, Ben Salem C. Drug-Induced Hyperglycaemia and Diabetes. Drug Saf [Internet]. 2015;38(12):1153-68. Available from: https://doi.org/10.1007/s40264-015-0339-z

[7] Thorell A, Rooyackers O, Myrenfors P, Soop M, Nygren J, Ljungqvist OH. Intensive insulin treatment in critically ill trauma patients normalizes glucose by reducing endogenous glucose production. J Clin Endocrinol Metab. 2004 Nov;89(11):5382-6.

[8] Inzucchi SE, Bergenstal RM, Buse JB, Diamant M, Ferrannini E, Nauck M, et al. Management of hyperglycemia in type 2 diabetes: A patient-centered approach. Diabetes Care. 2012;35(6):1364-79.

[9] Diabetes [Internet]. [cited 2021 Jun 20]. Available from: https://www.who.int/news-room/fact-sheets/detail/diabetes

[10] Kamenova P. Therapeutic potential of metformin in normal glucose tolerant persons with metabolic syndrome. Biotechnol Biotechnol Equip [Internet]. 2020;34(1):30-7. Available from: https://doi.org/10.1080/13102818.2019.1711184

[11] Hostalek U, Gwilt M, Hildemann S. Therapeutic Use of Metformin in Prediabetes and Diabetes Prevention. Drugs. 2015;75(10):1071-94.

[12] Marik PE, Bellomo R. Stress hyperglycemia: an essential survival response! Crit Care. 2013 Mar;17(2):305.

[13] Luna B, Feinglos MN. Drug-induced hyperglycemia. JAMA. 2001 Oct;286(16):1945-8.

[14] Tosur M, Viau-Colindres J, Astudillo M, Redondo MJ, Lyons SK. Medication-induced hyperglycemia: pediatric perspective. BMJ open diabetes Res care. 2020 Jan;8(1).

[15] Frontoni S, Picconi F. Impact of Drugs on Diabetes Risk and Glycemic Control. In 2019.

[16] Jain V, Patel RK, Kapadia Z, Galiveeti S, Banerji M, Hope L. Drugs and hyperglycemia: A practical guide. Maturitas. 2017 Oct;104:80-3.

[17] Byun DJ, Wolchok JD, Rosenberg LM, Girotra M. Cancer immunotherapy - immune checkpoint blockade and associated endocrinopathies. Nat Rev Endocrinol. 2017 Apr;13(4):195-207.

[18] de Filette JMK, Pen JJ, Decoster L, Vissers T, Bravenboer B, Van der

Auwera BJ, et al. Immune checkpoint inhibitors and type 1 diabetes mellitus: a case report and systematic review. Eur J Endocrinol. 2019 Sep;181(3):363-74.

[19] Smith AP, Banks J, Buchanan K, Cheong B, Gunawardena KA. Mechanisms of abnormal glucose metabolism during the treatment of acute severe asthma. Q J Med. 1992 Jan;82(297):71-80.

[20] Donihi AC, Raval D, Saul M, Korytkowski MT, DeVita MA. Prevalence and predictors of corticosteroid-related hyperglycemia in hospitalized patients. Endocr Pract [Internet]. 2006 Jul 1;12(4):358-62. Available from: https://doi.org/10.4158/EP.12.4.358

[21] Ochola LA, Nyamu DG, Guantai EM, Weru IW. Metformin's effectiveness in preventing prednisone-induced hyperglycemia in hematological cancers. J Oncol Pharm Pract [Internet]. 2019 Sep 7;26(4):823-34. Available from: https://doi.org/10.1177/10781552 19873048

[22] Henderson DC, Cagliero E, Gray C, Nasrallah RA, Hayden DL, Schoenfeld DA, et al. Clozapine, diabetes mellitus, weight gain, and lipid abnormalities: A five-year naturalistic study. Am J Psychiatry. 2000 Jun;157(6):975-81.

[23] Touger J. Introductory physics : building understanding. Diabetes Care. 2006;27(2):904.

[24] Abernathy E, Glaunsinger B. Since January 2020 Elsevier has created a COVID-19 resource centre with free information in English and Mandarin on the novel coronavirus COVID-19. The COVID-19 resource centre is hosted on Elsevier Connect, the company' s public news and information. 2020;(January).

[25] Pittas AG, Siegel RD, Lau J. Insulin therapy for critically ill hospitalized

patients: a meta-analysis of randomized controlled trials. Arch Intern Med. 2004 Oct;164(18):2005-11.

[26] Umpierrez GE, Hellman R, Korytkowski MT, Kosiborod M, Maynard GA, Montori VM, et al. Management of hyperglycemia in hospitalized patients in non-critical care setting: An endocrine society clinical practice guideline. J Clin Endocrinol Metab. 2012;97(1):16-38.

[27] Kodner C, Anderson L, Pohlgeers K. Glucose Management in Hospitalized Patients. Am Fam Physician. 2017;96(10):648-54.

[28] Umpierrez GE, Pasquel FJ. Management of inpatient hyperglycemia and diabetes in older adults. Diabetes Care. 2017;40(4):509-17.

[29] Magaji V, Johnston JM. Inpatient management of hyperglycemia and diabetes. Clin Diabetes. 2011;29(1):3-9.

[30] Lazar HL. Glycemic Control during Coronary Artery Bypass Graft Surgery. ISRN Cardiol. 2012;2012:1-14.

[31] Peng L, Smiley D, Newton C, Pasquel F, Fereira ME, Umpierrez G. Risk Factors for Inpatient Hypoglycemia during Subcutaneous Insulin. J Diabetes Sci Technol. 2012;6(5):1022-9.

[32] Handelsman Y, Henry RR, Bloomgarden ZT, Dagogo-Jack S, DeFronzo RA, Einhorn D, et al. American Association of Clinical Endocrinologists And American College of Endocriniology Position Statement On The Association Of SGLT-2 Inhibitors And Diabetic Ketoacidosis. Endocr Pract Off J Am Coll Endocrinol Am Assoc Clin Endocrinol. 2016 Jun;22(6):753-62.

[33] Standards of medical care in diabetes—2015 abridged for primary care providers. Clin Diabetes. 2015 Apr;33(2):97-111.

[34] Inzucchi SE, Bergenstal RM, Buse JB, Diamant M, Ferrannini E, Nauck M, et al. Management of Hyperglycemia in Type 2 Diabetes, 2015: A Patient-Centered Approach: Update to a position statement of the american diabetes association and the european association for the study of diabetes. Diabetes Care. 2015;38(1): 140-9.

[35] Ferlay J, Soerjomataram I, Dikshit R, Eser S, Mathers C, Rebelo M, et al. Cancer incidence and mortality worldwide: Sources, methods and major patterns in GLOBOCAN 2012. Int J Cancer. 2015;136(5):E359-86.

[36] Care H, Standards D. Diabetes care in the hospital. Diabetes Care. 2017;40(January):S120-7.

[37] Magalhães FO, Gouveia LMB, Torquato MTCG, Paccola GMGF, Piccinato CE, Foss MC. Metformin increases blood flow and forearm glucose uptake in a group of non-obese type 2 diabetes patients. Horm Metab Res = Horm und Stoffwechselforsch = Horm Metab. 2006 Aug;38(8): 513-7.

[38] Cusi K, Consoli A, DeFronzo RA. Metabolic effects of metformin on glucose and lactate metabolism in noninsulin-dependent diabetes mellitus. J Clin Endocrinol Metab. 1996 Nov;81(11):4059-67.

[39] Kamenova P, Atanasova I, Kirilov G. Metformin Improves Insulin Secretion and Reduces Insulin Resistance in People at High Risk for Development of Type 2 Diabetes Mellitus and Cardiovascular Disease. 2016;4(3):152-61.

[40] Panahi Y, Mojtahedzadeh M, Zekeri N, Beiraghdar F, Khajavi MR, Ahmadi A. Metformin treatment in hyperglycemic critically ill patients: Another challenge on the control of adverse outcomes. Iran J Pharm Res. 2011;10(4):913-9.

[41] An H, He L. Current understanding of metformin effect on the control of hyperglycemia in diabetes. J Endocrinol. 2016;228(3):R97-106.

[42] Viollet B, Guigas B, Sanz Garcia N, Leclerc J, Foretz M, Andreelli F. Cellular and molecular mechanisms of metformin: an overview. Clin Sci (Lond). 2012 Mar;122(6):253-70.

[43] Hardie DG, Ross FA, Hawley SA. AMPK: a nutrient and energy sensor that maintains energy homeostasis. Nat Rev Mol Cell Biol [Internet]. 2012;13(4):251-62. Available from: https://doi.org/10.1038/nrm3311

[44] Foretz M, Guigas B, Bertrand L, Pollak M, Viollet B. Review Metformin : From Mechanisms of Action to Therapies. Cell Metab [Internet]. 2014;20(6):953-66. Available from: http://dx.doi.org/10.1016/j.cmet.2014. 09.018

[45] El-Mir MY, Nogueira V, Fontaine E, Avéret N, Rigoulet M, Leverve X. Dimethylbiguanide inhibits cell respiration via an indirect effect targeted on the respiratory chain complex I. J Biol Chem. 2000;275(1): 223-8.

[46] Owen MR, Doran E, Halestrap AP. Evidence that metformin exerts its anti-diabetic effects through inhibition of complex 1 of the mitochondrial respiratory chain. Biochem J [Internet]. 2000 Jun 7;348(3):607-14. Available from: https://doi.org/10.1042/ bj3480607

[47] Duca FA, Côté CD, Rasmussen BA, Zadeh-Tahmasebi M, Rutter GA, Filippi BM, et al. Metformin activates a duodenal Ampk–dependent pathway to lower hepatic glucose production in rats. Nat Med [Internet]. 2015;21(5):506-11.

Available from: https://doi.
org/10.1038/nm.3787

[48] Christ-crain M, Kola B, Lolli F, Fekete C, Seboek D, Feltrin D, et al. AMP-activated protein kinase mediates glucocorticoid- induced metabolic changes : a novel mechanism in Cushing' s syndrome. 22(6):1672-83.

[49] Nader N, Sin S, Ng M, Lambrou GI, Pervanidou P, Wang Y, et al. AMPK Regulates Metabolic Actions of Glucocorticoids by Phosphorylating the Glucocorticoid Receptor through p38 MAPK. 2018;24(September 2010): 1748-64.

[50] Miller RA, Chu Q, Xie J, Foretz M, Viollet B, Birnbaum MJ. Biguanides suppress hepatic glucagon signalling by decreasing production of cyclic AMP. Nature. 2013 Feb;494(7436):256-60.

[51] Diabetes T, Program P. Prevention or delay of type 2 diabetes. Diabetes Care. 2017;40(January):S44-7.

[52] Karlsson HKR, Hällsten K, Björnholm M, Tsuchida H, Chibalin AY, Virtanen KA, et al. Effects of metformin and rosiglitazone treatment on insulin signaling and glucose uptake in patients with newly diagnosed type 2 diabetes: A randomized controlled study. Diabetes. 2005;54(5):1459-67.

[53] Bostrom B, Uppal P, Chu J, Messinger Y, Gandrud L, McEvoy R. Safety and efficacy of metformin for therapy-induced hyperglycemia in children with acute lymphoblastic leukemia. J Pediatr Hematol Oncol. 2013;35(7):504-8.

[54] Seelig E, Meyer S, Timper K, Nigro N, Bally M, Pernicova I, et al. Metformin prevents metabolic side effects during systemic glucocorticoid treatment. Eur J Endocrinol. 2017 Mar;176(3):349-58.

[55] Garber MD AJ, PhD, Duncan MD TG, Goodman MD AM, Mills RN DJ, BSN, et al. Efficacy of Metformin in Type II Diabetes. Am J Med [Internet]. 2018 Feb 6;103(6):491-7. Available from: http://dx.doi.org/10.1016/ S0002-9343(97)00254-4

[56] Sr S, Greyber E, Ga P, Ee S. Risk of fatal and nonfatal lactic acidosis with metformin use in type 2 diabetes mellitus (Review). 2010;(4).

[57] Nye HJ, Herrington WG. Metformin: The safest hypoglycaemic agent in chronic kidney disease? Nephron-Clin Pract. 2011;118(4):380-3.

[58] Pilmore HL. Review: Metformin: Potential benefits and use in chronic kidney disease. Nephrology. 2010;15(4): 412-8.

[59] Lipska KJ, Bailey CJ, Inzucchi SE. Use of metformin in the setting of mild-to-moderate renal insufficiency. Diabetes Care. 2011;34(6):1431-7.

[60] Davies MJ, D'Alessio DA, Fradkin J, Kernan WN, Mathieu C, Mingrone G, et al. Management of hyperglycemia in type 2 diabetes, 2018. A consensus report by the American Diabetes Association (ADA) and the european association for the study of diabetes (EASD). Diabetes Care. 2018;41(12):2669-701.

[61] Strack T. Metformin: a review. Drugs Today (Barc). 2008 Apr;44(4):303-14.

[62] Diabetes N, Clearinghouse I. Diabetes Prevention Program (DPP).

[63] Björkhem-Bergman L, Asplund AB, Lindh JD. Metformin for weight reduction in non-diabetic patients on antipsychotic drugs: a systematic review and meta-analysis. J Psychopharmacol. 2011 Mar;25(3):299-305.

[64] Temprosa M. Long-term effects of metformin on diabetes prevention:

Identification of subgroups that benefited most in the diabetes prevention program and diabetes prevention program outcomes study. Diabetes Care. 2019;42(4):601-8.

[65] Knowler WC, Barret-Connor E, Fowler SE, Hamman RF, Lachin JM, Walker EA, et al. Reduction in the Incidence of Type 2 Diabetes with Lifestyle Intervention or Metformin. N Engl J Med [Internet]. 2002;346(6):393-403. Available from: http://www.nejm.org/doi/abs/10.1056/NEJMoa012512

Section 2

Pharmacokinetics of Metformin

Chapter 3

Clinical Pharmacokinetics of Metformin

Tadesse Sheleme

Abstract

Metformin, the only biguanide oral antidiabetic agent available, was first used clinically in the late 1950s. Metformin remains the first-line pharmacologic treatment for type 2 diabetes patients. It can be used as a single agent or in combination therapy with other antidiabetes agents, including insulin. Metformin is absorbed predominately from the small intestine. It is rapidly distributed following absorption and does not bind to plasma proteins. It is excreted unchanged in urine. The elimination half-life of Metformin during multiple dosages in patients with good renal function is approximately 5 hours.

Keywords: metformin, clinical pharmacokinetics, type 2 diabetes

1. Introduction

Metformin is a biguanide developed from galegine, aguanidine derivative found in *Galega officinalis*. Chemically, it is a hydrophilic base which exists at physiological pH as the cationic species [1, 2]. Metformin is the first-line drug for type 2 diabetes and the most commonly prescribed drug for this condition worldwide, either alone or in combination with insulin or other oral antidiabetes patients [3]. Metformin works by inhibiting the production of hepatic glucose, reducing intestinal glucose absorption and improving glucose uptake and utilization. Besides lowering the blood glucose level, metformin may have additional health benefits, including weight reduction, lowering plasma lipid levels, and prevention of some vascular complications [4]. Metformin is also used for other indications such as polycystic ovary syndrome (PCOS) [5]. Metformin is increasingly recognized as a potential anticancer agent due to a reduced cancer incidence in diabetic patients treated with the drug, and recently, patients taking metformin were associated with a reduced risk of COVID-19-related mortality [6].

Metformin can be determined in biological fluids by various methods, mainly using high performance liquid chromatography (HPLC), which allows pharmacokinetic studies in healthy volunteers and diabetic patients. Metformin disposition is apparently unaffected by the presence of diabetes and only slightly affected by the use of different oral formulations [2]. The oral absorption, hepatic uptake and renal excretion of metformin are mediated very largely by organic cation transporters [7].

2. Absorption

Metformin is orally administered in the dose range of 500 mg/b.i.d. or t.i.d. and up to a total of 2,550 mg/day or approximately 35 mg/kg/day. The immediate-release formulation of metformin is rapidly absorbed from the small intestine following an oral dose. It has an onset of action of about 1.5 hours, half-life in the circulation of about 1.5–4.9 hours, and duration of action of 16–20 hours [8]. About 20% of a total dose can be absorbed from the duodenum, up to 60% from the jejunum and ileum but only very small amounts from the colon. The rest is excreted in the feces [9]. Higher doses slow the rate of absorption and reduce the bioavailability [10]. Oral absorption of metformin from the immediate-release dosage forms is incomplete in man, with an estimated population mean of 55% for bioavailability [6]. Metformin has an absolute oral bioavailability of 40 to 60%, and gastrointestinal absorption is apparently complete within 6 hours of ingestion [11]. Its hydrophilicity is associated with the low intestinal and cell membrane permeability, which is recognized as a primary limiting step for metformin oral absorption [6].

The extended-release formulation has a similar onset of effect; however, its half-life is 6.5 hours, and its duration of action is 24 hours. Therefore, it can be administered once daily. It is associated with fewer gastrointestinal side effects compared with the immediate-release formulation. The half-life of metformin may be prolonged in patients with renal impairment, resulting in a theoretical risk of the rare but fatal lactic acidosis. It has been suggested that this risk may be a consequence of the action of metformin to suppress gluconeogenesis resulting in the inhibition of lactic acid metabolism in the liver, and thus accumulation of lactate [8].

The intestinal absorption of metformin may be primarily mediated by plasma membrane monoamine transporter (PMAT). However, there is no in-vivo data which indicates the role of PMAT in the disposition and pharmacological effect of metformin [5].

3. Distribution

Metformin is rapidly distributed following absorption and does not bind to plasma proteins [11]. The volume of distribution has been reported to range from 63 to 276 L after intravenous administration [1]. The concentration of metformin in the liver is three to five fold higher than that in the portal vein (40–70 µmol/L) after single therapeutic dose (20 mg/kg/day in humans or 250 mg/kg/day in mice) [3, 8], and metformin in general circulation is 10–40 µmol/L [8]. As the antihyperglycemic effect of metformin is mainly due to the inhibition of hepatic glucose output and the concentration of metformin in the hepatocytes is much higher than in the blood, the liver is therefore presumed to be the primary site of metformin function [12]. At usual clinical doses and dosing schedules of metformin hydrochloride tablets, steady-state plasma concentrations of metformin are reached within 24 to 48 hours and are generally <1 mcg/mL [4].

4. Metabolism and elimination

Metformin is not metabolized and is excreted unchanged in the urine, with a half-life of ~5 hrs. The population mean for renal clearance (CLr) is 510±120 ml/min. Active tubular secretion in the kidney is the principal route of metformin elimination [5]. The total amount of metformin excreted under steady-state conditions with 1 g BID is around 6 mmol. The average feces volume is 150 ml per 24 hours; the calculated drug concentration in the distal colon is 40 mM. Not all of this may be free drug, as *E. coli* (with membrane potentials of −120 to −240 mV) may concentrate Metformin with subsequent block of its dihydrofolate reductase. The other 6 mmol reach the general circulation via the portal vein and, passing the liver, are rapidly cleared by the kidneys. The plasma elimination rate, about 500 ml per min, is similar to the kidney plasma flow, indicating active secretion [9].

The factors probably contribute to high clearance of metformin include: the low molecular weight associated with a negligible plasma protein binding; the presence of transporters in the kidney; and the low lipid solubility which makes negligible the passive reabsorption. The clearance is reduced in proportion to the reduction of renal function [13]. Metformin is contraindicated if serum creatinine levels ≥1.5 mg/dL in males, and ≥1.4 mg/dL in females or abnormal creatinine clearance. It should not be initiated in patients 80 years of age unless measurement of creatinine clearance demonstrates that renal function is not reduced [14].

5. Therapeutics range

The therapeutic range of plasma concentrations of metformin is unclear; however, concentrations above 5 mg/L are considered elevated [15]. Metformin immediate release (IR) taken BID and metformin extended release (XR), taken once daily (QD) in the evening with a meal, have almost equal areas under the curve (AUCs) for the same total dose. Both formulations have similar efficacy and safety profiles [9].

Metformin accumulation is a risk factor for fatal lactic acidosis. Therefore, therapeutic drug monitoring of metformin is required as an effort to ascertain that metformin concentration is within the recommended therapeutic range [16]. It is suggested that the mean plasma concentrations of metformin over a dosage interval be maintained below 2.5 mg/L in order to minimize the development of this adverse effect [7].

6. Therapeutics monitoring

Administration of ≥ 900 mg/kg/day of metformin resulted in morbidity/mortality and clinical signs of toxicity in rats. Increased incidence of minimal necrosis with minimal to slight inflammation of the parotid salivary gland for male rats given 1200 mg/kg/day, body weight loss and clinical signs in rats given ≥ 600 mg/kg/day were observed. Metformin was also associated with evidence of minimal metabolic acidosis at doses ≥ 600 mg/kg/day in rats [17]. In a preclinical study, intravenous and intragastric administration of metformin produced a significant increases in lactate AUC at the higher metformin doses (500 and 750 mg/kg), but intra-ileum administration did not produce an increase in lactate AUC relative to vehicle at either dose [18].

Large overdoses of metformin can lead to lactic acidosis. Suicide with metformin is rare. Intake of 35 g of metformin has been shown to be lethal [19]. The clinical study observed that patients on treatment with metformin developed lactic acidosis with metformin levels ranging from 256 to 682 μmol/L. This indicates that high levels of serum metformin are needed to cause lactic acidosis [20]. Metformin plasma levels >5 μg/mL are generally found when metformin is implicated as the cause of lactic acidosis [21]. Metformin plasma concentration levels do not exceed 5 μg/mL during controlled clinical trials, even at maximum doses [4]. Renal dysfunction, sepsis, alcohol abuse, liver failure, radiologic contrast media administration, acute coronary syndrome, acute congestive heart failure, and shock increase the risk of metformin-related lactic acidosis [22].

Metformin plasma concentrations are approximately 2–4 fold higher in patients with moderate to severe renal impairment [21]. According to the Food and Drug Administration (FDA) recommendation, metformin is contraindicated in patients with an estimated glomerular filtration (eGFR) <30 mL/min/1.73 m^2. Those with an eGFR between 30 and 45 mL/min/1.73 m^2 should not be initiated on metformin. If a person's eGFR falls between 30 and 45 mL/min/1.73 m^2 and they are already treated with metformin, their provider should assess their risk and benefit associated with continued use [22].

Elderly patients, who often have reduced muscle mass, should have their creatinine clearance rate estimated before use. If the creatinine clearance rate is < 70–80 ml/min, metformin should not be given [23]. Because hepatic function impairment may significantly limit the ability to clear lactate, generally avoid using metformin in patients with clinical or laboratory evidence of hepatic disease. Caution patients against excessive alcohol intake, either acute or chronic, when taking metformin because alcohol potentiates the effects of metformin on lactate metabolism [24].

Gastrointestinal intolerance occurs quite frequently in the form of abdominal pain, flatulence, and diarrhea. Most of these effects are transient and subside once the dose is reduced or when administered with meals. Metformin may reduce vitamin B12 absorption due to calcium-dependent ileal membrane antagonism, an effect that can be reversed with supplemental calcium. This vitamin B12 deficiency is rarely associated with megaloblastic anemia [25].

7. Drug interaction

Metformin is a cation at physiological pH, as it is a strong base. Hence, the absorption, distribution and excretion of Metformin depend on the transporters such as organic cation transporters, multidrug and toxin extruders and plasma membrane monoamine transporter [26]. The oral absorption and hepatic uptake of Metformin are mediated possibly by organic cation transporters-1 and -3 and renal excretion of Metformin is largely mediated by Metformin transporters such as multidrug and toxin extruders-1 and 2-k and organic cation transporter 2 [5]. The drugs inhibiting the Metformin transporters could decrease the elimination of Metformin and increase its plasma concentrations leading to elevated risk of Metformin associated lactic acidosis [27].

Since Metformin is not metabolized, it is not expected to be involved in many drug–drug interactions. Thus, clinically significant drug interactions involving metformin are rare [25]. Some cationic agents such as amiloride, digoxin, morphine, procainamide, quinidine, quinine, ranitidine, triamterene, trimethoprim, and vancomycin that are eliminated by renal tubular secretion may compete with metformin for elimination. Concomitant administration of cimetidine, furosemide, or nifedipine may also increase the concentration of metformin [23, 25].

The studies found many drugs which interact with metformin, but only a small number of clinically relevant drugs were identified which include cimetidine, contrast agents, dolutegravir, phenprocoumon, pyrimethamine, ranolazine, rifampicin, St John's wort, trimethoprim, vandetanib and verapamil (**Table 1**) [26]. Verapamil remarkably decreases the glucose-lowering effect of metformin, without altering its pharmacokinetics. This is likely mediated by competitive

Medication	Mechanism of interaction	Consequences/effects	Recommendation
Cimetidine	Elimination It competes with metformin for renal elimination and decreases the excretion of metformin.	It increases exposure of Metformin and risk of Metformin associated lactic acidosis.	It is recommended to reduce the dose of Metformin when Cimetidine is co-prescribed.
Trimethoprim	It inhibits Metformin elimination moderately through the inhibition of OCTs and MATEs.	It decreases Metformin clearance and increases plasma concentration.	Monitor carefully in patients with renal dysfunction or patients taking higher doses of Metformin
Rifampin	Absorption The mechanism may involve rifampin-mediated induction of the OCT1 in the gastrointestinal tract.	Rifampin may increase the gastrointestinal absorption and therapeutic efficacy of metformin.	Close clinical monitoring of glycemic control is recommended, and the dosage of metformin may be adjusted as necessary.
Dolutegravir	It is an inhibitor of both OCT2 and MATE1 transporters within the renal tubules.	It may increase the risk of hypoglycemia and GI intolerance due to increased plasma concentrations of Metformin.	Prescribers may adjust the Metformin dose to prevent intolerable adverse effects while prescribing both drugs.
Pyrimethamine	Elimination It decreases renal clearance of Metformin by the inhibition of OCT2 and MATE transporters.	Co-administration of Pyrimethamine with Metformin results in elevated plasma concentrations Metformin.	Metformin dose adjustment should be considered.
Ranolazine	Elimination It may decrease the Metformin elimination through the inhibition of OCT2 transporter.	The plasma concentration of Metformin is elevated by the co-administration of Ranolazine.	This interaction is dose dependent and it is recommended that the daily dose of Metformin should not exceed 1700 mg in patients taking Ranolazine 1000 mg two times daily.
Vandetanib	Elimination Vandetanib is a potent inhibitor of MATE1 and MATE2K transporters.	Its co-administration with Metformin may result in increased plasma concentration of Metformin due to decreased elimination.	The patients receiving both drugs should be monitored carefully for Metformin toxicity.

OCT- Organic cation transporter; MATEs-Multidrug and toxin extruders; GI-Gastrointestinal

Table 1.
Clinically a significant pharmacokinetic drug interactions of metformin.

inhibition of organic cation transporter 1 [28]. Metformin should be discontinued at least 48 hours prior to the administration of iodinated contrast media which can produce acute renal failure and should only be restarted if renal function is normal [25]. Study observed that Metformin decreases the anticoagulant effect of phenprocoumon [29].

8. Conclusion

Metformin is widely used for the treatment of type 2 diabetes mellitus. Metformin is a highly ionized, water-soluble drug that is absorbed, distributed and eliminated by transporters [15]. It undergoes active tubular secretion in the kidney and is excreted unchanged in the urine. A change in pharmacokinetics can alter drug exposure and predispose the patient to either over- or under dosing, potentially resulting in adverse drug reactions or therapeutic failure [30]. Most of the possible drug interactions of Metformin occur through the inhibition of organic cation transporter and multidrug and toxin extruders and increase the risk of Metformin associated lactic acidosis. Metformin administration should be stopped and urgent medical attention given to the patients developing first signs of lactic acidosis such as severe vomiting and diarrhea [27].

Author details

Tadesse Sheleme
Department of Pharmacy, College of Health Science, Mettu University, Mettu, Ethiopia

*Address all correspondence to: tadeshe14@gmail.com

IntechOpen

References

[1] Graham GG, Punt J, Arora M, Day RO, Doogue MP, Duong JK, et al. Clinical pharmacokinetics of metformin. Clin Pharmacokinet. 2011;50(2):81-98.

[2] Scheen AJ. Clinical pharmacokinetics of metformin. Clinical pharmacokinetics. 1996;30(5):359-371.

[3] Flory J, Lipska K. Metformin in 2019. Jama. 2019;321(19):1926-1927.

[4] Dumitrescu R, Mehedintu C, Briceag I, Purcărea V, Hudita D. Metformin-clinical pharmacology in PCOs. Journal of medicine and life. 2015;8(2):187.

[5] Gong L, Goswami S, Giacomini KM, Altman RB, Klein TE. Metformin pathways: Pharmacokinetics and pharmacodynamics. Pharmacogenetics and genomics. 2012;22(11):820.

[6] Jeong Y-S, Jusko WJ. Meta-assessment of metformin absorption and disposition pharmacokinetics in nine species. Pharmaceuticals. 2021;14(6):545.

[7] Graham GG, Punt J, Arora M, Day RO, Doogue MP, Duong J, et al. Clinical pharmacokinetics of metformin. Clinical pharmacokinetics. 2011;50(2):81-98.

[8] Apampa B. Pharmacology and safe prescribing of metformin. Nurse Prescribing. 2012;10(12):597-602.

[9] Glossmann HH, Lutz OM. Pharmacology of metformin—An update. European journal of pharmacology. 2019;865:172782.

[10] Kinaan M, Ding H, Triggle CR. Metformin: An old drug for the treatment of diabetes but a new drug for the protection of the endothelium. Medical principles and practice. 2015;24(5):401-415.

[11] Scheen AJ. Clinical pharmacokinetics of metformin. Clin Pharmacokinet. 1996;30(5):359-371.

[12] Song R. Mechanism of metformin: A tale of two sites. Diabetes care. 2016;39(2):187-189.

[13] Vecchio S, Giampreti A, Petrolini V, Lonati D, Protti A, Papa P, et al. Metformin accumulation: Lactic acidosis and high plasmatic metformin levels in a retrospective case series of 66 patients on chronic therapy. Clinical Toxicology. 2014;52(2):129-135.

[14] Inzucchi SE, Lipska KJ, Mayo H, Bailey CJ, McGuire DK. Metformin in patients with type 2 diabetes and kidney disease: A systematic review. Jama. 2014;312(24):2668-2675.

[15] Duong JK, Kumar SS, Kirkpatrick CM, Greenup LC, Arora M, Lee TC, et al. Population pharmacokinetics of metformin in healthy subjects and patients with type 2 diabetes mellitus: Simulation of doses according to renal function. Clinical pharmacokinetics. 2013;52(5):373-384.

[16] Wibowo A, Ningrum VD, Izzah N, editors. Stability Test of Metformin Hydrochloride in Human Plasma Using HPLC-UV for the Protocol of Therapeutic Drug Monitoring of Metformin. AIP Conference Proceedings; 2018: AIP Publishing LLC.

[17] Quaile MP, Melich DH, Jordan HL, Nold JB, Chism JP, Polli JW, et al. Toxicity and toxicokinetics of metformin in rats. Toxicology and applied pharmacology. 2010;243(3):340-347.

[18] Bailey C, Wilcock C, Scarpello J. Metformin and the intestine. Diabetologia. 2008;51(8):1552-1553.

[19] Gjedde S, Christiansen A, Pedersen SB, Rungby J. Survival

following a metformin overdose of 63 g: A case report. Pharmacology and toxicology. 2003;93(2):98-99.

[20] Anders Frid M, Sterner GN, Löndahl M, Wiklander C, Cato A, Ellen Vinge M, et al. Novel assay of metformin levels in patients with type 2 diabetes and varying levels of renal function. Diabetes Care. 2010;33(6):1291.

[21] DeFronzo R, Fleming GA, Chen K, Bicsak TA. Metformin-associated lactic acidosis: Current perspectives on causes and risk. Metabolism. 2016;65(2):20-29.

[22] Wooley AC, Kerr JL. Monitoring patients on metformin: Recent changes and rationales. Journal of Pharmacy Technology. 2018;34(1):28-36.

[23] Triplitt C. Drug interactions of medications commonly used in diabetes. Diabetes Spectrum. 2006;19(4):202-211.

[24] Crowley MJ, Diamantidis CJ, McDuffie JR, Cameron B, Stanifer J, Mock CK, et al. Metformin use in patients with historical contraindications or precautions. 2017.

[25] Rojas LBA, Gomes MB. Metformin: An old but still the best treatment for type 2 diabetes. Diabetology and metabolic syndrome. 2013;5(1):1-15.

[26] Stage TB, Brøsen K, Christensen MMH. A comprehensive review of drug–drug interactions with metformin. Clinical pharmacokinetics. 2015;54(8):811-824.

[27] Maideen NMP, Jumale A, Balasubramaniam R. Drug interactions of metformin involving drug transporter proteins. Advanced pharmaceutical bulletin. 2017;7(4):501.

[28] Cho SK, Kim CO, Park ES, Chung JY. Verapamil decreases the glucose-lowering effect of metformin in healthy volunteers. British journal of clinical pharmacology. 2014;78(6):1426-1432.

[29] Wijnen J, Van de Riet I, Lijfering W, Van der Meer F. Metformin use decreases the anticoagulant effect of phenprocoumon. Journal of Thrombosis and Haemostasis. 2014;12(6):887-890.

[30] Roberts DM, Sevastos J, Carland JE, Stocker SL, Lea-Henry TN. Clinical pharmacokinetics in kidney disease: Application to rational design of dosing regimens. Clinical Journal of the American Society of Nephrology. 2018;13(8):1254-1263.

Uses, Adverse Drug Reactions and Drug Interactions of Metformin

Chapter 4

Metformin: Pros and Cons

Shalini Sivadasan, Muthukumar Subramanian and
Rajasekaran Aiyalu

Abstract

Metformin was approved for the treatment of Type 2 Diabetes Mellitus in 1958 for UK, in 1972 for Canada and in 1995 by FDA in USA. Metformin is the drug of choice for patients who are obese and have type 2 diabetes mellitus. Though metformin was at first proven to treat hyperglycemia, many other uses of metformin are proven to be effective. It is also used for gestational diabetes mellitus, obesity, hyper secretion of ovarian androgen, poly-cystic ovary syndrome (PCOS), anti-psychotic therapy induced weight gain, cancer treatment and anti-aging. Metformin causes a decrease in appetite thus known to act on obesity. The other action of metformin is reduction of circulating levels of insulin and insulin like growth factor 1 (IGF-1) which is associated with anticancer action. There are ongoing researches about the effect of metformin on anti-aging properties and proved that metformin is linked with anti-aging factors. Three main factors that are related with aging are oxidation, glaciation and methylation. Metformin as all drugs, have unwanted effects as well. Many side effects of metformin are considered mild where lactic acidosis and vitamin B12 deficiency happens to be the major.

Keywords: metformin uses, diabetes mellitus, obesity, poly-cystic ovary syndrome, cancer

1. Introduction

1.1 Pros (uses) of metformin

Metformin, the most common drug used to treat type 2 diabetes, approved by U.S. Food Drug Administration (US-FDA) (1), belongs to a class of drugs called biguanides with a guanidine and galegine connection. Metformin was approved for treatment of Type 2 Diabetes Mellitus in 1958 for UK [1], 1972 for Canada [2] and 1995 by FDA in USA [1, 3].

Metformin (1,1-dimethyl biguanide hydrochloride) was synthesized in 1920's. Since then, the drug became the first choice to treat type 2 diabetes due to its remarkable ability to decrease plasma glucose levels [4–6]. It acts by reducing the glucose made by liver, decreasing the amount glucose that body absorbs and increasing the effect of insulin in the body [7].

In recent years, studies have shown many unexpected effective roles of metformin that exerts strong effect on cardiovascular disease (CVD) [8], cancers [9, 10], neurodegenerative diseases [11], liver diseases [12], obesity [13, 14], and renal diseases [15], hypersecretion of ovarian androgens, poly-cystic ovary syndrome (PCOS), anti-psychotic therapy induced weight gain, and anti-aging [16].

The agent also offers neuro protection that may reduce the risk of dementia and stroke [17].

1.1.1 Metformin in diabetes

Several studies and clinical trials have confirmed that metformin mono therapy or combination therapy with other glucose-lowering drugs is successful in treating type 2 diabetes. Metformin is the drug of choice for diabetic patients who are obese and have type 2 diabetes mellitus.

Type 2 diabetes coexists with insulin resistance and leads to extremely high blood sugar levels. Metformin lowers blood sugar, preventing permanent organ damage, which in due course could lead to dysfunction and failure [18, 19]. Metformin exerts its anti-hyperglycemic effects through AMP which initiates the uptake of sugar from the blood into muscles.

Metformin exerts its anti-hyperglycemic effects by suppressing hepatic glucose production through AMPK dependent [20, 21] or -independent pathways [22, 23].

Metformin increases AMPK that leads to more sugar being taken from the blood into tissues, thus lowering the blood sugar level [24].

It is used in case of insulin resistance as it works by decreasing hepatic glucose production, decreasing peripheral insulin resistance and improving insulin sensitivity thereby increasing peripheral glucose uptake and utilization. Metformin does not produce hypoglycaemia and does not cause hyperinsulinemia in normal patients or in patients with type 2 diabetes. Insulin secretion remains unchanged whereas fasting insulin levels and daylong plasma insulin response may decrease with metformin therapy [25].

On the other hand, metformin may reduce blood sugar by inhibiting the production of new glucose (gluconeogenesis) from non-carbohydrates such as lactate, glycerol, and some amino acids [23]. Metformin inhibits gluconeogenesis through AMPK-dependent activation of small hetero dimer partner (SHP) and inhibition of phosphorylation of CREB binding protein (CBP) [26], thereby suppressing the expression of gluconeogenic genes, such as G6Pase (glucose 6 phosphatase), PEPCK (phosphoenolpyruvate carboxykinase), and PC (pyruvate carboxylase) [27].

Studies also suggest that metformin could enhance GLUT1 (glucose transporter 1) mediated glucose transport into hepatocytes by activating IRS2 (insulin receptor substrate two), decreasing plasma glucose levels [28].

Besides decreasing liver glucose production, metformin also decreases glucose levels through increasing (i) GLUT4 (glucose transporter 4) mediated glucose uptake in skeletal muscles [29] and (ii) absorption of glucose in the intestines [30]. Metformin also stimulates glucagon-like-peptide-1 (GLP-1) release, thereby improving insulin secretion and reducing plasma glucose levels [31]. The molecular mechanism of metformin in hepatic gluconeogenesis and glucose production is shown in **Figure 1**.

A clinical trial conducted on over 3,000 people who were at risk of developing type 2 diabetes showed that those people treated with metformin had a 31% lower occurrence of type 2 diabetes compared to the placebo group [34].

1.1.2 Metformin in gestational diabetes

Gestational diabetes mellitus (GDM) is the most common medical complication of pregnancy which is associated with insulin resistance (IR) and hyperinsulinemia that may predispose some women to develop diabetes. Gestational diabetes has been defined as any degree of glucose intolerance with an onset, or first recognition during pregnancy [35]. In 2013, the World Health Organization (WHO) recommended

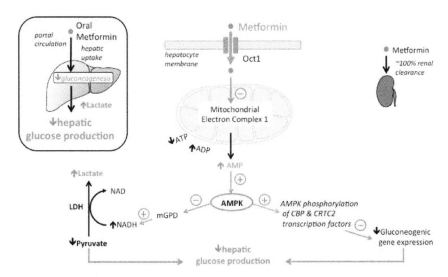

Figure 1.
Metformin in hepatic gluconeogenesis and glucose production. Metformin acts primarily to suppress glucose production in the liver. While metformin's mechanism(s) of action remain controversial, current evidence indicates that metformin's most important effect in treating diabetes is to lower the hepatic production of glucose [32, 33].

that hyperglycemia first detected during pregnancy be classified as either 'diabetes mellitus (DM) in pregnancy' or 'GDM' [36]. GDM is associated with short- and long-term sequelae on both, mother and offspring [37, 38].

During normal pregnancy, around the mid-pregnancy, a progressive insulin resistance develops that progresses during the third trimester. In early pregnancy, insulin secretion increases, while insulin sensitivity remain unchanged, decreased or increased whereas in mid pregnancy, insulin sensitivity declines progressively and worsens during the rest of the pregnancy, being worst in the late third trimester, which rebounds with the delivery of the placenta. Therefore, GDM usually develops in the late second trimester and disappears, instantly, post-delivery [39].

For GDM, lifestyle interventions such as daily exercise, medical nutrition therapy is the initial treatment while, metformin, the oral hypoglycemic agent is being considered as a substitute to insulin. The rationale behind using metformin in gestational and pre-existing diabetes during pregnancy is as metformin increases insulin sensitivity, reduces hepatic glucogeneogenesis and enhances peripheral glucose uptake, resulting in lowering of blood glucose with minimal risk of maternal hypoglycemia and weight gain [40].

Although, metformin has been shown to pass freely across the placenta [41], there are no reported adverse side effects to the fetus when it is used to treat women with infertility caused by poly-cystic ovary syndrome (PCOS) [42, 43]. Metformin is classified as a category B drug, which implies that there is no confirmation of animal or fetal toxicity or teratogenicity. The study of metformin in pregnancy revealed that the use of metformin in women with GDM was not associated with increased risk of congenital anomalies, or maternal and neonatal complications compared to insulin, except for higher rates of preterm labour [44].

Results of systematic review and meta-analysis had shown that metformin is better than insulin in reducing, maternal weight gain during pregnancy and the frequency of pregnancy induced hypertension, with no changes in the frequency of hypoglycemia and pre-eclampsia [45]. In addition, randomized controlled trials (RCT) suggest that metformin could be used to treat or prevent pre-eclampsia [46]. Metformin is considered as the first-line drug in the management of type 2 diabetes due to its efficacy, tolerability and safety in non-pregnant individuals.

1.1.3 Metformin in polycystic ovary syndrome

Poly-cystic ovarian syndrome (PCOS) is a hormonal disorder often aggravated by obesity and insulin resistance. PCOS is an endocrine-metabolic dysfunction among 5–10% of women in reproductive age which is associated with metabolic disturbances that have a high impact in cardio metabolic diseases, such as insulin resistance [47–49].

PCOS is characterized by menstrual irregularities, low fertility, obesity and high blood levels of male hormones in reproductive aged women [50]. PCOS confirms insulin resistance which leads to the hypothesis of a pre-diabetic state with glucose intolerance, gestational diabetes mellitus and evident diabetes. Several studies show that insulin resistance stimulates the ovaries to produce male hormones, i.e., androgens. This causes stigmata of androgen excess such as hirsutism and acne. Metformin increases insulin sensitivity and decreases the production of ovarian androgen thereby normalizing the hormone levels, stabilizes menstrual irregularities and improves fertility and ovulation. It also directly inhibits the androgen production [51].

Metformin treats PCOS symptoms, such as irregular ovulation or menstrual cycles, and the excess of insulin in the body. It has also been made known to treat PCOS symptoms by reducing body mass index (BMI) and testosterone levels. Furthermore, metformin assists fertility and increases the chance of successful pregnancy and reduces the risk of early miscarriage, gestational diabetes, and inflammation associated with PCOS. Metformin is thus used as the drug of choice for the treatment of PCOS. More to that, metformin helps mothers carry their baby to full term [51, 52]. Metformin is strongly recommended in patients with metabolic syndrome and obesity [51].

1.1.4 Metformin in obesity

Obesity is a chronic disease accompanied with metabolic syndromes, such as diabetes, fatty liver diseases, and cardiovascular diseases (CVDs). Obesity is caused by an imbalance between energy intake and expenditure [53].

Metformin happens to be one of the drugs available for the treatment of obesity. Metformin acts on obesity by decreasing the appetite and reduced BMI levels. Metformin contains a primary anorectic factor which reduces the appetite. Leptin levels were found to be decreased on taking metformin. Moreover, glucagon like peptide-1 levels rise significantly on taking metformin. This promotes weight loss. It was observed that adults with severe obesity lost weight more significantly than mildly obese patients [54]. Metformin exerts its anti-obesity effects through increasing mitochondrial biogenesis, decreasing fatty acid uptake, and stimulating thermogenesis [55].

It acts by promoting sugar dysplasia restrains and reducing inhibition caused by insulin-induced expression of the glucose transporter protein, thus increasing glucose utilization [56]. Metformin is effective in reducing body weight and improving insulin sensitivity in adults, and is used to treat adolescents who are overweight or obese and unresponsive to changes in lifestyle or who present with insulin resistance [57]. Many studies support that metformin can promote weight loss in overweight or obesity patients [58, 59]. Based on the reports it is understood that clinical trials supports the efficacy and safety profiles of metformin in diabetes and weight gain prevention [60].

1.1.5 Metformin in medication induced weight gain

Studies have shown that use of antipsychotics increase the risk of weight gain, dyslipidemia and diabetes. Weight gain and abdominal adiposity which is directly associated with insulin resistance, dyslipidemia and risk of diabetes may be induced by second generation antipsychotics [61, 62]. Stimulation of appetite, reducing physical activity and impairing metabolic regulation is the mechanism of antipsychotics induced weight gain [63].

Metformin aids in weight loss. Drug induced weight gain can be reduced by metformin. It assists in reduction of weight for those who gain 10% of body weight than pre-treatment [63]. Metformin contains an anorectic factor and facilitates less hunger. This also aids in decreased appetite. Metformin causes decreased leptin levels, thus suppresses appetite. Metformin also increases the GLP-1 levels which enhances weight loss. Thus, metformin with lifestyle changes is effective in the treatment of weight gain induced by antipsychotics.

1.1.6 Metformin in cancer

New studies have shown that metformin is effective in killing cancer cells. In trials, people undergoing chemotherapy alone saw their cancer return, while for those on chemo and metformin, their tumors disappeared. Research has shown that those taking metformin are less likely to develop certain cancers. Metformin has been found to improve cancer prognosis as it inhibits cancer cell growth and proliferation. Evidence points that metformin inhibits growth, survival, and metastasis of different types of tumor cells, including those from breast, liver, bone, pancreas, endometrial, colorectal, kidney, and lung cancers [64].

Metformin prevented the growth and spreading of certain cancers in patients with type 2 diabetes. This proposed mechanism is through a known tumor-suppressant gene (LKB1), which activates AMPK. Metformin shows anticancer properties by direct and indirect regulation of cells' metabolism. The direct effects are mediated by AMPK dependent and -independent pathways. (i) Metformin activates AMPK, which leads to the inhibition of mTOR signaling, and thereby disturbs the protein synthesis, and suppresses the cell growth and proliferation [65]. As an antidiabetic drug, metformin decreases plasma glucose levels, thereby inhibiting cancer cell proliferation and survival [66].

Other studies reported that metformin could activate the immune response against cancer cells [67] or decrease NF-kB (nuclear factor-kB) activity, which results in a reduction in the secretion of pro-inflammatory cytokines [68].

Metformin activates AMPK and then induces p53 phosphorylation to prevent cell invasion and metastasis [69].

The different mechanisms antitumor action has been proposed which involves the following: (a) the activation of adenosine monophosphate kinase, (b) modulation of adenosine A1 receptor (ADORA), (c) reduction in insulin/insulin growth factors, and (d) inhibition of endogenous reactive oxygen species (ROS); and its resultant damage to deoxyribonucleic acid (DNA) molecule is another paramount antitumor mechanism [70].

Metformin reduces the proliferation of cancer cells and the possibility of malignancies in different types of cancer, including gastric carcinoma, pancreatic cancer, uterine cancer, medullary thyroid cancer [71]. **Figure 2** shows the mechanism of metformin in Cancer and **Figure 3** shows the direct and indirect effects of metformin in Cancer.

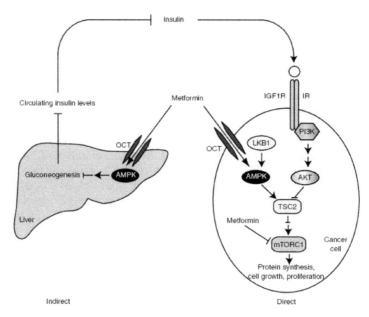

Figure 2.
Mechanism of metformin in Cancer. The anticancer activity of metformin is associated with direct and indirect effects of the drug. The direct insulin-independent effects of metformin are mediated by activation of AMPK and a reduction in mTOR signaling and protein synthesis in cancer cells [72].

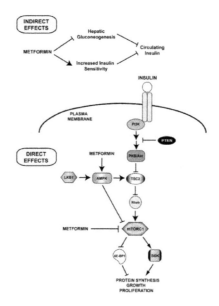

Figure 3.
Direct and indirect effects of metformin on cancer. Metformin activates AMPK leading to stabilization of TSC2 and inhibition of mTORC1 signaling and protein synthesis. Metformin can also directly target mTOR independently of AMPK and TSC2 [73].

1.1.6.1 Breast cancer

Breast cancer (BC) is one of the most common malignancies occurring in females. Cellular glucose metabolism is linked tightly with the proliferation and development of breast cancer. Several studies suggested that metformin reduces the incidence of breast cancer in type 2 diabetes patients [74]. Cancer cells show enhanced glucose uptake and metabolism and prefer glycolysis. The noted specialty of metformin is to decrease glucose levels, thereby limiting the availability of energy for cancer cells. Metformin decreases FAS expression which is an essential component of the fatty acid synthesis pathway, therefore affecting the survival of cancer cells.

1.1.6.2 Blood cancer

Leukemia comprises 2.8% of all cancers and 3.4% of cancer-related deaths world-wide. The aberrant activation of the PI3K/AKT/mTOR pathway is one of the most common biochemical features of leukemia [75]. Metformin inhibits AKT/mTOR signaling, which is an effective approach to treat leukemia. Metformin plays a beneficial role in human lymphoma by inhibiting mTOR signaling without the involvement of AKT, and the suppression of mTOR subsequently leads to the suppression of growth of B cells and T cells [76].

1.1.6.3 Colorectal cancer (CRC)

CRC is also one of the most common cancers in the world. In 2004, relationship between metformin and CRC was demonstrated [77]. Metformin may exert its pharmacodynamic effects through the gut-brain-liver axis, but these mechanisms require further exploration. In the intestine, metformin increases glucose uptake and lactate concentrations. Administration of metformin increases the bile acid pool in the intestine that may affect GLP-1 secretion and cholesterol levels. In addition, metformin changes the microbiome, affecting the regulation of metabolism, such as glucose homeostasis, lipid metabolism, and energy metabolism [78]. These changes inhibits the development and progress of CRC.

1.1.6.4 Bone cancers

Compared with cancers initiating in bone tissue itself, invasion of metastatic cancers, especially breast, lung, and prostate cancers, into bones is more common [79]. All types of bone cancers influence the osteolytic process, and osteoblastic metastases occur through osteoclast activation or stimulant factors which are responsible for osteoblastic proliferation, differentiation, and formation [80].

1.1.6.5 Endometrial cancer

Metabolic syndrome like obesity and hyperglycemia is related to the development of endometrial cancer. Metformin is an effective anti-diabetic drug, studies have demonstrated the beneficial effect of metformin on endometrial cancer development by the mechanisms involving the mitochondrial OXPHOS suppression and AMPK activation which subsequently inhibit a variety of metabolic pathways, including STAT3, ZEB-1, ACC, mTOR, and IGF-1 [81].

1.1.6.6 Melanoma

Melanoma is the most aggressive skin cancer and is responsible for almost 80% of the skin cancer-related deaths. Due to its strong invasive ability, melanoma often metastasizes to the lymph nodes, liver, lungs, and even the central nervous system [82]. Metformin can induce cell cycle arrest in the G0–G1 phase in melanoma cells. Another study indicated that metformin can attenuate melanoma growth and metastasis through inhibiting the expression of TRB3 (tribbles pseudokinase 3) in non-diabetic and diabetic mouse models [83]. Because of the activation effect of AMPK, metformin could influence melanoma cell death and proliferation and the tumor microenvironment. It will be interesting to investigate the effects of combination treatment of metformin with current therapies or other drugs to treat melanoma.

1.1.7 Metformin in aging

Aging is considered unavoidable and is modulated by genetic and dietary factors. The declining ability to regenerate damaged tissue and the deterioration in homeostatic processes are considered as biological features of aging [84]. Usually, the primary causes foraging are DNA damage and autophagy. Aging is a result of DNA damage, which can be induced by ROS, alkylation, hydrolysis, chemicals, and ultraviolet and other radiation [85]. Trials have shown metformin's efficacy in reducing the effects of aging, such as decreasing age-related illnesses, problems with cognitive function, and morbidity [86].

Metformin slows down aging and reduces the incidence of aging-related diseases such as neurodegenerative disease and cancer in humans. In spite of its widespread use, the mechanisms by which metformin exerts favorable effects on aging remain largely unknown [87]. The mechanisms by which metformin affects the aging process are partly dependent on the regulation of glucose metabolism. By inhibiting mitochondrial complex I, metformin reduces endogenous production of ROS and subsequently decreases DNA damage [88].

By activating AMPK, metformin is able to inhibit NF-kB signaling and attenuate cell inflammation [89]. Metformin also leads to decreased insulin levels, and suppresses IGF-1 signaling and mTOR signaling, resulting in suppression of inflammation and autophagy, which is beneficial to the aging process [90]. Besides, metformin was shown to have a function in the regulation of the microbiome, which may be another way to affect aging [91]. There are three main factors that are related with aging. They are oxidation, glycation and methylation. There is evidence that metformin acts as an anti-aging agent. It helps slow the rate of aging and retain youth characteristics for a longer period of time than compared to non-metformin users. There are ongoing research about the effect of metformin on anti-aging properties. Researches have proved that metformin is linked with anti-aging factors [92].

There are two mechanisms to describe aging. First one is ROS theory, i.e., reactive oxygen species [93]. The ROS theory explains that by products of oxidative phosphorylation are reactive oxygen species, i.e., free radicals. The free radicals increase significantly and damage other cells and organs. The ROS leads to DNA damage [64].

The second mechanism is TOR theory. Cellular pathway like IGF-1 axis, MAPK, AKT, PI3K stimulated by mitogens, growth factors, sugars and amino acids are said to inhibit aging. Caloric restriction suppresses the mTOR pathway. The activity of mTOR may be inhibited by rapamycin. Rapamycin has gero-suppressive effects. These include extending the lifespan, prevent age related disorders and reduce cost of patient care. AMPK activation led to an indirect inhibition of mTOR. Metformin acts as an AMPK activator [64, 94]. Metformin, Being an AMPK activator, metformin has been proved to have gero-suppressive effects. Extended longevity and lifespan were seen in those taking metformin. Autophagy plays a significant role in gero-suppressive mechanisms. Autophagy protects cell organelles and nutrient supply. Induction of autophagy extends the lifespan. Polyamines cause autophagy. Activation of autophagy induces processes associated with suppression of IGF and mTOR pathways. Therefore metformin acts as an activator of autophagy [95].

1.1.8 Metformin in liver diseases

Liver dysfunction may lead to many diseases, such as diabetes, non-alcoholic fatty liver disease, cirrhosis, non-alcoholic hepatitis, and hepatocellular carcinoma. Studies showed that metformin is safe in patients with cirrhosis. In diabetic patients, metformin caused a 50% reduction in hepatocellular carcinoma incidence and improved survival mainly by influencing cell growth and angiogenesis through the PI3K/AKT/mTOR signaling pathway [96]. In humans, metformin was also found to reduce the incidence of fatty liver diseases and to cause a histological response [97]. However, other studies showed that metformin failed to improve liver histology, hepatic steatosis, and inflammation [98].

1.1.9 Metformin and cardiovascular diseases

Hyperglycemia induces oxidative stress, resulting in lipoprotein dysfunction and endothelial dysfunction, increasing the risk of CVD. Metformin was shown to decrease the incidence of CVD in diabetes patients. Metformin was also shown to decrease irregular heartbeats and lower oxidative stress [86]. Through activating AMPK, metformin inhibits alpha-dicarbonyl-mediated modification of apolipoprotein residues, consequently ameliorating high density lipoprotein (HDL) dysfunction and reducing low density lipoprotein (LDL) modifications. Reductions in HDL dysfunction improve cholesterol transport and diminish the cardiovascular risk. Moreover, metformin improves endothelial oxidative stress levels and attenuates hyperglycemia-induced inflammation, decreasing the occurrence of CVD [99]. It has been shown that metformin improves the myocardial energy status through ameliorating cellular lipid and glucose metabolism via AMPK [100].

1.1.10 Metformin and renal diseases

Diabetes is considered as an important cause of renal diseases, and metformin is an interesting candidate to treat renal diseases, although its use was restricted previously [101]. Daily oral administration of metformin could improve kidney fibrosis and normalize kidney structure and function. These effects may be mediated by the AMPK signaling pathway, which can regulate cell growth and energy utilization. Another study found that in a CKD mouse model, metformin could suppress kidney injury and improve kidney function, through AMPK-mediated ACC signaling [102].

It is worth to note that appropriate dosage of metformin is very important in the treatment for renal diseases. The mechanisms underlying these kidney protective roles of metformin may be related to the regulation of glucose utilization, the decrease in cell inflammation, and oxidative stress [103]. The summary of metformin in different diseases and the underlying major mechanism is shown in the **Figure 4.**

1.2 Cons (side effects) of metformin

Metformin as all drugs, have unwanted effects which can be mild or serious side effects. The most common side effects are related to gut complications and include upset stomach, nausea, vomiting, diarrhea, light headedness, or a metallic taste in the mouth [104]. In general, older patients may be at an increased risk for some of its side effects, such as lactic acidosis or low blood sugar, due to other factors [104]. The minor side effects include gastrointestinal disturbances. The most common are anorexia, nausea, abdominal discomfort and diarrhea. Dose reduction or discontinuation of the drug may reduce or alleviate these symptoms. Out of the side effects,

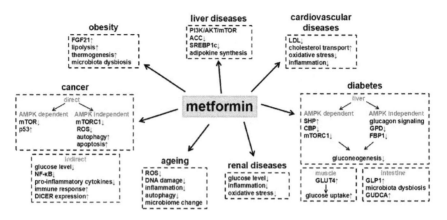

Figure 4.
Summary of metformin in different diseases and the underlying major mechanism [103].

lactic acidosis and vitamin B12 deficiency happens to be the major. Although rare, if lactic acidosis occurs, may be fatal, which may occur in presence of hypoxia and renal insufficiency [105].

1.2.1 Lactic acidosis

Lactic acidosis is a condition in which lactic acid builds up in the body, altering pH balance and potentially leading to complications [106]. Because metformin reduces the breakdown of lactate to glucose, the drug may induce lactic acidosis if it accumulates significantly. Metformin's exact mechanism of action in doing so is unknown. More frequently, the combination of this drug and an underlying health condition may trigger lactic acidosis [107].

The rate of developing lactic acidosis increases in patients with predisposing factors, such as renal impairment, hepatic disease, congestive heart failure or sepsis. Metformin is renally cleared. In cases of renal failure or decreased creatinine clearance, metformin accumulates. When this happens, it inhibits mitochondrial electron transport. Therefore, it increases anerobic metabolism and lactic production [108]. The levels of lactate increase in metformin taking patients. The pyruvate dehydrogenase inhibits conversion of lactate to glucose, thereby causes lactic acidosis [109].

Because metformin decreases liver uptake of lactate, any condition that may precipitate lactic acidosis is a contraindication. Patients with infections, recent surgery, kidney or liver damage, history of heart disease, respiratory failure, excessive alcohol consumption (due to depletion of NAD+ stores), or dehydration have an increased risk of lactic acidosis induced by metformin [110]. The FDA recommends avoiding the use of metformin in more severe chronic kidney disease, below the eGFR cutoff of 30 ml/minute/1.73 m^2.

Lactate uptake by the liver is diminished with metformin use because lactate is a substrate for hepatic gluconeogenesis, a process that metformin inhibits. Metformin-associated lactate production may also take place in the large intestine, which could potentially contribute to lactic acidosis in those with risk factors. Elderly patients are also at risk for developing lactic acidosis [104, 111].

1.2.2 Vitamin B12 deficiency

A common report with long term metformin use is vitamin B12 malabsorption which leads to vitamin B12 deficiency [112, 113]. With increased metformin dosage, the incidence of vitamin B12 deficiency also increased [114]. In a study, it was proven that being treated with metformin had a 7% greater risk of vitamin B12 deficiency than with placebo [115].

The mechanisms leading to vitamin B12 deficiency may be explained by changes in small intestine motility. This cause increased bacterial growth and hence, consumption of vitamin B12. Metformin also inhibits the calcium dependent absorption of vitamin B12 [116]. Vitamin B12 is an essential nutrient for cognitive and cardiovascular function [117, 118]. Clinical manifestations of vitamin B12 deficiency include alteration in mental status, megaloblastic anemia and neurological damage [118].

1.2.3 Hypoglycemia

Metformin, itself, does not lead to a state of critically low blood sugar. In combination with other risk factors such as heavy alcohol drinking (or dehydration), the use of other drugs for diabetes, insufficient calorie intake, or bouts of heavy exercise, it may increase the chances of developing hypoglycemia [100]. Since metformin does not directly stimulate insulin secretion, hypoglycemia risk may be lower than for that of other oral anti-diabetes drugs. However, hypoglycemia in patients using metformin may occur in association with strenuous physical activity or fasting [119].

1.2.4 Anemia

Metformin can decrease the levels of vitamin B12 in our body. In rare cases, this can cause anemia or low levels of red blood cells. Metformin use is associated with early risk of anemia in individuals with type 2 diabetes. The mechanism for this early fall in hemoglobin is uncertain, but given the time course, is unlikely to be due to vitamin B_{12} deficiency alone [120].

Vitamin B12 (cobalamin) deficiency is a frequent cause of megaloblastic anemia that is evident through various symptoms [121]. However, the mechanism for these findings is unclear. Because development of anemia was not obviously associated with a rising mean cell volume (MCV) or macrocytosis, vitamin B12 deficiency is an unlikely explanation in most cases. We should evaluate anemia in metformin users as we would for any patient; if a thorough evaluation is unrevealing, we might cautiously attribute the anemia to metformin [120].

1.2.5 Cognitive impairments

A case–control study of over 7,000 patients with Alzheimer's disease showed that, compared to insulin treatments, sulfonylureas, and thiazolidinediones, metformin was associated with an increased incidence of Alzheimer's [122]. However, another study on approximately 1,500 people showed that the cognitive impairment associated with metformin may be alleviated with vitamin B12 and calcium supplements [123]. Controversies are seen as studies have reported that metformin was found to significantly reduce the occurrence of cognitive dysfunction in patients with T2D [124]. Several studies found that metformin improved cognitive abilities [125, 126]. The relationship between metformin and cognitive dysfunction in patients with T2D is controversial.

1.2.6 Gastrointestinal

Gastrointestinal upset is most common when metformin is first administered, or when the dose is increased. This can cause severe discomfort which can often be avoided by starting the drug at a low dose and increasing the dose gradually, but even with low doses, 5% of people may be unable to tolerate metformin. Long-term use of metformin has been associated with increased homocysteine levels and malabsorption of vitamin B12. Higher doses and prolonged use are associated with increased incidence of vitamin B12 deficiency.

2. Conclusion

Metformin, the drug initially approved and used for the treatment of Type 2 diabetes mellitus is proven to be effective in many other conditions such as gestational diabetes mellitus, obesity, hypersecretion of ovarian androgens, poly-cystic ovary syndrome (PCOS), anti-psychotic therapy induced weight gain, cancer treatment etc. There are ongoing research about the effect of metformin on anti-aging properties and proved that metformin is linked with anti-aging factors.

Author details

Shalini Sivadasan*, Muthukumar Subramanian and Rajasekaran Aiyalu
KMCH College of Pharmacy, Coimbatore, Tamil Nadu, India

*Address all correspondence to: shaliniravichandran11@gmail.com

IntechOpen

References

[1] Bailey CJ. Metformin: historical overview. Diabetologia 2017; 60: 1566-1576. doi: 10.1007/s00125-017-4318-z.

[2] Lucis OJ. The status of metformin in Canada. Canadian Medical Association Journal. 1983; 128(1):24-26.

[3] DeFronzo RA, Goodman AM, Multicenter Metformin Study Group. Efficacy of metformin in patients with non-insulin-dependent diabetes mellitus. N Engl J Med. 1995; 333: 541-549.

[4] Witters LA. The blooming of the French lilac. J Clin Invest. 2001; 108:1105– 7. doi: 10.1172/JCI14178.

[5] Papanagnou P, Stivarou T, Tsironi M. Unexploited antineo plastic effects of commercially available anti-diabetic drugs. Pharmaceuticals. 2016: 9:24. doi: 10.3390/ph9020024.

[6] Blonde L, Dipp S, Cadena D. Combination glucose-lowering therapy plans in T2DM: case-based considerations. Adv Ther. 2018; 35:939-965. doi: 10.1007/s12325-018-0694-0.

[7] Metformin, oral tablet. 2018; Available at https://www.medicalnewstoday.com/articles/metformin-oral-tablet#interactions.

[8] Lamanna C, Monami M, Marchionni N, Mannucci E. Effect of metformin on cardiovascular events and mortality: a meta-analysis of randomized clinical trials. Diabetes Obes Metab. 2011; 13:221-228. doi: 10.1111/j.1463-1326.2010.01349.x.

[9] Gandini S, Puntoni M, Heckman-Stoddard BM, Dunn BK, Ford L, Decensi A, et al. Metformin and cancer risk and mortality: a systematic review and meta-analysis taking into account biases and confounders. Cancer Prev Res. 2014; 7:867-885. doi: 10.1158/1940-6207.CAPR-13-0424.

[10] Morales DR, Morris AD. Metformin in cancer treatment and prevention. Annu Rev Med. 2015; 66:17-29. doi: 10.1146/annurev-med-062613-093128.

[11] Patrone C, Eriksson O, Lindholm D. Diabetes drugs and neurological disorders: new views and therapeutic possibilities. Lancet Diabetes Endocrinol. 2014; 2:256-262. doi: 10.1016/S2213-8587(13)70125-6.

[12] Bhat A, Sebastiani G, Bhat M. Systematic review: preventive and therapeutic applications of metformin in liver disease. World J Hepatol. 2015; 7:1652-1659. doi: 10.4254/wjh.v7.i12.1652.

[13] Breining P, Jensen JB, Sundelin EI, Gormsen LC, Jakobsen S, Busk M, et al. Metformin targets brown adipose tissue in vivo and reduces oxygen consumption in vitro. Diabetes Obes Metab. 2018; 20:2264-2273. doi: 10.1111/dom.13362.

[14] Bannister CA , Holden SE, Jenkins-Jones S, Morgan CL, Halcox JP, Schernthaner G, Mukherjee J, Currie CJ. Can people with type 2 diabetes live longer than those without? A comparison of mortality in people initiated with metformin or sulphonylurea monotherapy and matched, non-diabetic controls. Diabetes Obes Metab. 2014; 16(11):1165-1173. doi: 10.1111/dom.12354.

[15] Neven E, Vervaet B, Brand K, Gottwald-Hostalek U, Opdebeeck B, De Mare A, et al. Metformin prevents the development of severe chronic kidney disease and its associated mineral and bone disorder. Kidney Int. 2018; 94:102-113. doi: 10.1016/j.kint.2018.01.027

[16] Non-Diabetic Uses of Metformin. Available at http://oureverydaylife.com/

nondiabetic-uses-metformin-11813. htm. Accessed on May 23, 2017.

[17] Ng TP, Feng L, Yap KB, Lee TS, Tan CH, Winblad B. Long-term metformin usage and cognitive function among older adults with diabetes. J Alzheimers Dis. 2014; 41(1):61-68. doi: 10.3233/JAD-131901.

[18] Alam U, Asghar O, Azmi S , Malik RA. General aspects of diabetes mellitus. Handb Clin Neurol. 2014; 126:211-222. doi: 10.1016/B978-0-444-53480-4.00015-1.

[19] Bailey CJ, Turner RC. Metformin. N Engl J Med. 1996; 334(9):574-579. doi: 10.1056/NEJM199602293340906.

[20] Shaw RJ, Lamia KA, Vasquez D, Koo SH, Bardeesy N, Depinho RA, et al. The kinase LKB1 mediates glucose homeostasis in liver and therapeutic effects of metformin. Science. 2005; 310:1642-1646. doi: 10.1126/science. 1120781.

[21] Fullerton MD, Galic S, Marcinko K, Sikkema S, Pulinilkunnil T, Chen ZP, et al. Single phosphorylation sites in Acc1 and Acc2 regulate lipid homeostasis and the insulin-sensitizing effects of metformin. Nat Med. 2013; 19:1649-1654. doi: 10.1038/nm.3372.

[22] Foretz M, Hebrard S, Leclerc J, Zarrinpashneh E, Soty M, Mithieux G, et al. Metformin inhibits hepatic gluconeogenesis in mice independently of the LKB1/AMPK pathway via a decrease in hepatic energy state. J Clin Invest. 2010; 120:2355-2369. doi: 10.1172/JCI40671.

[23] Madiraju AK, Erion DM, Rahimi Y, Zhang XM, Braddock DT, Albright RA, Prigaro BJ, Wood JL, Bhanot S, MacDonald MJ, Jurczak MJ, Camporez JP, Lee HY, Cline GW, Samuel VT, Kibbey RG, Shulman GI. Metformin suppresses gluconeogenesis by inhibiting mitochondrial glycerophosphate dehydrogenase. Nature. 2014; 510(7506):542-546. doi: 10.1038/nature13270.

[24] Gaochao Zhou, Robert Myers, Ying Li, Yuli Chen, Xiaolan Shen, Judy Fenyk-Melody, Margaret Wu, John Ventre, Thomas Doebber, Nobuharu Fujii, Nicolas Musi, Michael F. Hirshman, Laurie J. Goodyear, and David E. Moller. Role of AMP-activated protein kinase in mechanism of metformin action. J Clin Invest. 2001; 108(8):1167-1174. https://doi. org/10.1172/JCI13505.

[25] Dumitrescu R, Mehedintu C, Briceag I, Purcarea VL, and Hudita D. Metformin-Clinical Pharmacology in PCOs. J Med Life. 2015; 8(2): 187-192.

[26] He L, Sabet A, Djedjos S, Miller R, Sun X, Hussain MA, et al. Metformin and insulin suppress hepatic gluconeogenesis through phosphorylation of CREB binding protein. Cell. 2009; 137:635-646. doi: 10.1016/j.cell.2009.03.016.

[27] Herzig S, Long F, Jhala US, Hedrick S, Quinn R, Bauer A, et al. CREB regulates hepatic gluconeogenesis through the coactivator PGC-1. Nature. 2001; 413:179-183. doi: 10.1038/35093131.

[28] Gunton JE, Delhanty PJ, Takahashi S, Baxter RC. Metformin rapidly increases insulin receptor activation in human liver and signals preferentially through insulin-receptor substrate-2. J Clin Endocrinol Metab. 2003; 88:1323-1332. doi: 10.1210/ jc.2002-021394.

[29] Kristensen JM, Treebak JT, Schjerling P, Goodyear L, Wojtaszewski JF. Two weeks of metformin treatment induces AMPK-dependent enhancement of insulin-stimulated glucose uptake in mouse soleus muscle. Am J Physiol Endocrinol

Metab. 2014; 306:E1099–E1109. doi: 10.1152/ajpendo.004 17.2013.

[30] Gu S, Shi J, Tang Z, Sawhney M, Hu H, Shi L, et al. Comparison of glucose lowering effect of metformin and acarbose in type 2 diabetes mellitus: a metaanalysis. PLoS ONE. 2015; 10:e0126704. doi: 10.1371/journal.pone.0126704.

[31] Emilie Bahne, Emily W. L. Sun, Richard L. Young, Morten Hansen, David P. Sonne, Jakob S. Hansen, Ulrich Rohde, Alice P. Liou, Margaret L. Jackson, Dayan de Fontgalland, Philippa Rabbitt, Paul Hollington, Luigi Sposato, Steven Due, David A. Wattchow, Jens F. Rehfeld, Jens J. Holst, Damien J. Keating, Tina Vilsbøll, and Filip K. Knop. Metformin-induced glucagon-like peptide-1 secretion contributes to the actions of metformin in type 2 diabetes. JCI Insight. 2018; 3(23): e93936.

[32] He L, Wondisford FE. Metformin action: concentration matters. Cell Metab. 2015; 21(2):159-162. doi: 10.1016/j.cmet.2015.01.003

[33] Nolte Kennedy MS, Masharani U: Pancreatic Hormones & Antidiabetic Drugs (Chapter 41). In: *Basic & Clinical Pharmacology*. 15th Ed. Katzung BG, Trevor AJ (Editors). McGraw-Hill / Lange.2015

[34] Diabetes Prevention Program Research Group. Reduction In The Incidence Of Type 2 Diabetes With Lifestyle Intervention Or Metformin. N Engl J Med. 2002; 346(6):393-403. doi: 10.1056/NEJMoa012512.

[35] Classification and diagnosis of diabetes mellitus and other categories of glucose intolerance. National Diabetes Data Group. Diabetes. 1979; (12):1039-1057.

[36] World Health Organization. Diagnostic criteria and classification of hyperglycaemia first detected in pregnancy. Geneva (CH): World Health Organization; 2013. Available from: http: //130.14.29.110/books/NBK169024.

[37] Dall, T. M., Yang, W., Halder, P., Pang, B., Massoudi, M., Wintfeld, N., et al. The economic burden of elevated blood glucose levels in 2012: diagnosed and undiagnosed diabetes, gestational diabetes mellitus, and prediabetes. Diabetes Care. 2014; 37(12):3172-3179. doi: 10.2337/dc14-1036.

[38] Farrar, D., Simmonds, M., Bryant, M., Sheldon, T. A., Tuffnell, D., Golder, S., et al. Treatments for gestational diabetes: a systematic review and meta-analysis. BMJ Open. 2017; 7(6):e015557. doi: 10.1136/bmjopen-2016-015557.

[39] Catalano PM, Tyzbir ED, Roman NM, Amini SB, Sims EA. Longitudinal changes in insulin release and insulin resistance in nonobese pregnant women. Am J Obstet Gynecol. 1991; 165:1667-1672.

[40] Rena G, Hardie DG, Pearson ER. The mechanisms of action of metformin.Diabetologia. 2017; 60(9):1577-1585.

[41] Eyal S, Easterling TR, Carr D, Umans JG, Miodovnik M, Hankins GD, Clark SM, Risler L, Wang J, Kelly EJ, Shen DD, Hebert MF. Pharmacokinetics of metformin during pregnancy. Drug Metab Dispos. 2010; 38(5):833-840.

[42] Nawaz FH, Khalid R, Naru T, Rizvi J. Does continuous use of metformin throughout pregnancy improve pregnancy outcomes in women with polycystic ovarian syndrome? J Obstet Gynaecol Res. 2008; 34(5): 832-837.

[43] Bolton S, Cleary B, Walsh J, Dempsey E, Turner MJ. Continuation of metformin in the first trimester of women with polycystic ovarian syndrome is not associated with

increased perinatal morbidity. Eur J Pediatr. 2009; 168(2):203-206.

[44] Rowan JA, Hague WM, Gao W, Battin MR, Moore MP, MiG Trial Investigators. Metformin versus insulin for the treatment of gestational diabetes. N Engl J Med. 2008; 358(19):2003-2015.

[45] Gui, J, Liu Q, Feng L. Metformin vs insulin in the management of gestational diabetes: a meta-analysis. PloS One. 2013; 8(5), e64585. doi: 10.1371/journal.pone.0064585.

[46] Romero R., Erez O, Huttemann M, Maymon E, Panaitescu B, Conde-Agudelo A, et al. Metformin, the aspirin of the 21st century: its role in gestational diabetes mellitus, prevention of preeclampsia and cancer, and the promotion of longevity. Am. J. Obstet. Gynecol. 2017; 217 (3): 282-302. doi: 10.1016/j.ajog.2017.06.003.

[47] Dunaif A, Segal KR., Futterweit W, Dobrjansky A. Profound peripheral insulin resistance, independent of obesity, in polycystic ovary syndrome. Diabetes. 1989; 38 (9), 1165-1174. doi: 10.2337/diab.38.9.1165.

[48] Franks S. Polycystic ovary syndrome. N. Engl. J. Med. 1995; 333(13): 853-861. doi: 10.1056/ NEJM199509283331307.

[49] Holte, J. Disturbances in insulin secretion and sensitivity in women with the polycystic ovary syndrome. Baillieres Clin. Endocrinol. Metab. 1996; 10(2): 221-247. doi: 10.1016/ S0950-351X(96)80085-1.

[50] Lathief S and Pal L. Advances in Treatment options for Polycystic Ovarian Syndrome. Female Endocrinology. US Endocrinology. 2012; 8(1):57-64.

[51] Hsin-Shih W. The Role of Metformin in the Treatment of Polycystic Ovarian

Syndrome (PCOS). Forum. Chang Gung Med J. 2006; 29(5):445-447.

[52] Spritzer PM. PCOS: Reviewing Diagnosis and Management of Metabolic Disturbances. Arq Bras Endocrinal Metab. 2014; 58 (2): 182-187.

[53] Despres JP, Lemieux I. Abdominal obesity and metabolic syndrome. Nature. 2006; 444:881-887. doi: 10.1038/ nature05488.

[54] Aa MP, Hoving V, Garde EMW, Boer A, Knibbe CAT, Vorst MMJ. The Effect of Eighteen- Month Metformin Treatment in Obese Adolscents: Comparison of Results Obtained in Daily Practice with Results from a Clinical Trial. Journal of Obesity. 2016; 2016: 1-7.

[55] Karise I, Bargut TC, Del Sol M, Aguila MB, Mandarim-De-Lacerda CA. Metformin enhances mitochondrial biogenesis and thermogenesis in brown adipocytes of mice. Biomed Pharmacother. 2019; 111:1156-1165. doi: 10.1016/j.biopha.2019.01.021.

[56] Kirpichnikov D, McFarlane SI, Sowers JR. Metformin: an update. Ann Intern Med. 2002; 137:25-33.

[57] Caprio S. Treatment of impaired glucose tolerance in childhood. Nat Clin Pract Endocrinol Metab 2008; 4:320-332;

[58] McDonagh MS, Selph S, Ozpinar A, Foley C. Systematic review of the benefits and risks of metformin in treating obesity in children aged 18 years and younger. JAMA Pediatr. 2014; 168(2):178-184.

[59] Graff SK, Mario FM, Ziegelmann P, Spritzer PM. Effects of orlistat vs. metformin on weight loss-related clinical variables in women with PCOS: systematic review and meta-analysis. Int J Clin Pract. 2016; 70(6):450-461.

[60] Hostalek U, Gwilt M, Hildemann S. Therapeutic Use of Metformin in Prediabetes and Diabetes Prevention. Drugs. 2015; 75(10):1071-1094.

[61] Fenton WS and Chavez MR. Medication Induced Weight Gain and Dyslipidemia in Patients with Schizophrenia. Am J Psychiatry. 2016; 163(10): 1697-1704.

[62] Generali JA and Cada DJ. Off- Label Drug Uses, Metformin: Prevention and Treatment of Antipsychotic-Induced Weight Gain. Hosp Pharm. 2013; 48(9): 734-735.

[63] Fenton WS and Chavez MR. Medication Induced Weight Gain and Dyslipidemia in Patients with Schizophrenia. Am J Psychiatry. 2016; 163(10): 1697-1704.

[64] Podhorecka M, Ibanez B, Dmoszynska A. Metformin – its potential anticancer and anti-aging effects. Postepy Hig, Medycyny Doswiadczalnej. 2017; 71: 170-175. doi: 10.5604/01.3001.0010.3801.

[65] Gwinn DM, Shackelford DB, Egan DF, MihaylovaMM, Mery A, Vasquez DS, et al. AMPK phosphorylation of raptor mediates a metabolic checkpoint.Mol Cell. 2008; 30:214-226. doi: 10.1016/j. molcel.2008.03.003.

[66] Sui X, Xu Y, Wang X, Han W, Pan H, Xiao M. Metformin: a novel but controversial drug in cancer prevention and treatment. Mol Pharm. (2015) 12:3783-3791. doi: 10.1021/acs. molpharmaceut.5b00577.

[67] Pryor R, Cabreiro F. Repurposing metformin: an old drug with new tricks in its binding pockets. Biochem J. 2015; 471:307-322. doi: 10.1042/BJ20150497.

[68] MoiseevaO, Deschenes-Simard X, St-Germain E, Igelmann S, HuotG, Cadar AE, et al. Metformin inhibits the senescence-associated secretory phenotype by interfering with IKK/ NF-kappaB activation. Aging Cell. (2013) 12:489-98, doi: 10.1111/ acel.12075.

[69] Cerezo M, Tichet M, Abbe P, Ohanna M, Lehraiki A, Rouaud F, et al. Metformin blocks melanoma invasion and metastasis development in AMPK/ p53-dependent manner. Mol Cancer Ther. 2013; 12:1605-1615. doi: 10.1158/1535-7163.MCT-12-1226-T.

[70] Ugwueze CV, Ogamba OJ, Young EE, Onyenekwe BM and Ezeokpo BC. Metformin: A Possible Option in Cancer Chemotherapy. Analytical Cellular Pathology. 2020; https://doi.org/10.1155/2020/7180923.

[71] Rego DF, Pavan LM, Elias ST, De Luca Canto G, Guerra EN. Effects of metformin on head and neck cancer: a systematic review. Oral Oncol. 2015; 51(5):416-422.

[72] Kasznicki J, Sliwinska A, Drzewoski J. Metformin in cancer prevention and therapy. Ann Transl Med. 2014; 2:57. doi: 10.3978/j. issn.2305-5839.2014.06.01.

[73] Dowling R, Niraula S, Stambolic V, Goodwin P. Metformin in cancer: translational challenges. Journal of molecular endocrinology 2012; DOI:10.1530/JME-12-007

[74] Dowling RJ, Goodwin PJ, Stambolic V. Understanding the benefit of metformin use in cancer treatment. BMC Med 9: 33. Available at http:// www.biomedcentral.com/1741-7015/ 9/33

[75] Polak R, Buitenhuis M. The PI3K/ PKB signaling module as key regulator of hematopoiesis: implications for therapeutic strategies in leukemia. Blood. 2012; 119:911-923. doi: 10.1182/ blood-2011-07-366203.

[76] Shi WY, Xiao D, Wang L, Dong LH, Yan ZX, Shen ZX, et al. Therapeutic metformin/AMPK activation blocked lymphoma cell growth via inhibition of mTOR pathway and induction of autophagy. Cell Death Dis. 2012; 3:e275. doi: 10.1038/cddis.2012.13.

[77] Yang YX, Hennessy S, Lewis JD. Insulin therapy and colorectal cancer risk among type 2 diabetes mellitus patients. Gastroenterology. 2004; 127:1044-1050. doi: 10.1053/j. gastro.2004.07.011.

[78] Mccreight LJ, Bailey CJ, Pearson ER. Metformin and the gastrointestinal tract. Diabetologia. 2016; 59:426-435. doi: 10.1007/s00125-015-3844-9.

[79] Linnard-Palmer L. The use of simulation for pediatric oncology nursing safety principles: ensuring competent practice through the use of a mnemonic, chemotherapy road maps and case-based learning. J Pediatr Nurs. 2012; 27:283-286. doi: 10.1016/j. pedn.2012.02.001.

[80] Mundy GR. Metastasis to bone: causes, consequences and therapeutic opportunities. Nat Rev Cancer. 2002; 2:584-593. doi: 10.1038/nrc867.

[81] Ko EM, Walter P, Jackson A, Clark L, Franasiak J, Bolac C, et al. Metformin is associated with improved survival in endometrial cancer. Gynecol Oncol. 2014; 132:438-442. doi: 10.1016/j. ygyno.2013.11.021.

[82] Demierre MF. Epidemiology and prevention of cutaneous melanoma. Curr Treat Options Oncol. 2006; 7:181-186. doi: 10.1007/ s11864-006-0011-z.

[83] Li K, Zhang TT, Wang F, Cui B, Zhao CX, Yu JJ, et al. Metformin suppresses melanoma progression by inhibiting KAT5-mediated SMAD3 acetylation, transcriptional activity and TRIB3 expression. Oncogene. 2018;

37:2967-2981. doi: 10.1038/ s41388-018-0172-9.

[84] Losordo DW, Henry TD. New definition of aging? Measuring regenerative capacity in patients. Circ Res. 2016; 119:774-775. doi: 10.1161/ CIRCRESAHA.116.309622.

[85] Hoeijmakers JH. DNA damage, aging, and cancer. N Engl J Med. 2009; 361:1475-1485. doi: 10.1056/ NEJMra0804615.

[86] https://diabeticnation. com/2019/07/30/7-metformin-uses.

[87] Soukas AA, Hao H, Wu L. Metformin as Anti-Aging Therapy: Is It for Everyone? Trends Endocrinol Metab. 2019; 30(10):745-755. doi: 10.1016/j. tem.2019.07.015.

[88] Algire C, Moiseeva O, Deschenes-Simard X, Amrein L, Petruccelli L, Birman E, et al. Metformin reduces endogenous reactive oxygen species and associated DNA damage. Cancer Prev Res. 2012; 5:536-543.doi: 10.1158/1940-6207. CAPR-11-0536.

[89] Valencia WM, Palacio A, Tamariz L, Florez H. Metformin and ageing: improving ageing outcomes beyond glycaemic control. Diabetologia. 2017; 60:1630-1638. doi: 10.1007/ s00125-017-4349-5.

[90] Song YM, Lee YH, Kim JW, Ham DS, Kang ES, Cha BS, et al. Metformin alleviates hepatosteatosis by restoring SIRT1-mediated autophagy induction via an AMP-activated protein kinase-independent pathway. Autophagy. 2015; 11:46-59. doi: 10.4161/15548627.2014.984271.

[91] Barzilai N, Crandall JP, Kritchevsky SB, EspelandMA. Metformin as a tool to target aging. Cell Metab. 2016; 23:1060-1065. doi: 10.1016/j.cmet.2016.05.011.

[92] Arora BP. Anti-aging Medicine. Indian J. Plastic Surgery Supplement. 2008; 41: S130-S133.

[93] Foretz M, Guigas B, Bertrand L, Pollak M, Viollet B. Metformin: From Mechanism of Action to Therapies. Cell Metabolism 20. 2014; 20(6):953-966.

[94] Hawley SA, Gadalla AE, Olsen GS, Hardie DG. The Antidiabetic Drug Metformin Activates the AMP-Activated Protein Kinase Cascade via an Adenine Nucleotide- Independent Mechanism. Diabetes. 2002; 51: 2420-2425.

[95] Menendez JA, Cufi S, Oliveras-Ferraros C, Vellon L, Joven J, Vazquez-Martin A. Gerosuppressant Metformin: less is more. Aging. 2011; 3(4): 348- 362.

[96] Singh S, Singh PP, Singh AG, Murad MH, Sanchez W. Anti-diabetic medications and the risk of hepatocellular cancer: a systematic review and meta-analysis. Am J Gastroenterol. 2013; 108:881-891. doi: 10.1038/ajg.2013.5.

[97] Lavine JE, Schwimmer JB, Van Natta ML, Molleston JP, Murray KF, Rosenthal P, et al. Effect of vitamin E or metformin for treatment of nonalcoholic fatty liver disease in children and adolescents: the TONIC randomized controlled trial. JAMA. 2011; 305:1659-1668. doi: 10.1001/jama.2011.520.

[98] Tiikkainen M, Hakkinen AM, Korsheninnikova E, Nyman T, Makimattila S, Yki-Jarvinen H. Effects of rosiglitazone and metformin on liver fat content, hepatic insulin resistance, insulin clearance, and gene expression in adipose tissue in patients with type 2 diabetes. Diabetes. 2004; 53:2169-2176. doi: 10.2337/diabetes.53.8.2169.

[99] Kheniser KG, Kashyap SR, Kasumov T. A systematic review: the appraisal of the effects of metformin on lipoprotein modification and function. Obes Sci Pract. 2019; 5:36-45. doi: 10.1002/osp4.309.

[100] Dziubak A, Wojcicka G, Wojtak A, Beltowski J. Metabolic effects of metformin in the failing heart. Int J Mol Sci. 2018; 19:2869. doi: 10.3390/ijms19102869.

[101] Misbin RI, Green L, Stadel BV, Gueriguian JL, Gubbi A, Fleming GA. Lactic acidosis in patients with diabetes treated with metformin. N Engl J Med. 1998; 338:265-266. doi: 10.1056/NEJM199801223380415.

[102] Lee M, Katerelos M, Gleich K, Galic S, Kemp BE, Mount PF, et al. Phosphorylation of Acetyl-CoA Carboxylase by AMPK Reduces Renal Fibrosis and Is Essential for the Anti-Fibrotic Effect of Metformin. J Am Soc Nephrol. 2018; 29:2326-36. doi: 0.1681/ASN.2018010050.

[103] Lv Z and Guo Y (2020) Metformin and Its Benefits for Various Diseases. Front. Endocrinol. 2020; 11:191. doi: 10.3389/fendo.2020.00191.

[104] Hamid Nasri and Mahmoud Rafieian-Kopaei. Metformin: Current knowledge. J Res Med Sci. 2014; 19(7):658-664.

[105] Suh S. Metformin- Associated Lactic Acidosis. Endocrinology Metabolism. 2015; 30:45-46.

[106] Jeffrey KA and Nicolaos EM. Lactic acidosis. The New England journal of medicine, 371(24): 2309-2319. Doi.10.1056/nejmra1309483.

[107] Lalau JD, Kajbaf F, Protti A, Christensen MM, De Broe ME, Wiernsperger N. Metformin-associated lactic acidosis (MALA): Moving towards a new paradigm. Diabetes Obes Metab. 2017; 19(11):1502-1512. doi: 10.1111/dom.12974.

[108] Misbin RI. The Phantom of Lactic Acidosis due to Metformin in Patients with Diabetes. Diabetes Care. 2004; 27(7):1791-1793.

[109] Renda F, Mura P, Finco G, Ferrazin F, Pani L, Landoni G. Metformin- Associated Lactic Acidosis Requiring Hospitalization. A National 10 year Survey and a Systematic Literature Review. European Review for Medical and Pharmacological Sciences. 2013; 17(Supplement 1):45-49.

[110] Yazdi P. 9 Proven Metformin Uses + Side Effects. 2020; Available at https://selfhacked.com/blog/uses-benefits-metformin/#Side_Effects_of_Metformin. Accessed on 20 June 2021.

[111] Scheen AJ, Paquot N. Metformin revisited: a critical review of the benefit-risk balance in at-risk patients with type 2 diabetes. Diabetes Metab. 2013; 39(3):179-190. doi: 10.1016/j.diabet.2013.02.006.

[112] Kumthekar AA, Gidwani HV, Kumthekar AB. Metformin Associated B12 deficiency. JAPI. 2012; 60: 58-59.

[113] Kang D, Yun JS, Ko SH, Lim TS, Ahn YB, Park YM, Ko HS. Higher Prevalence of Metformin-Induced Vitamin B12 Deficiency in Sulfonylurea Compared with Insulin Combination in Patients with Type 2 Diabetes: A Cross- Sectional Study. PLoS ONE. 2014; 9(10):1-9.

[114] Liu Q, Li S, Quan H, Li J. Vitamin B12 status in metformin treated patients: systematic review. PLoS One. 2014; 9(6):e100379. doi: 10.1371/journal.pone.0100379.

[115] Jager J, Kooy A, Lehert P, Wulffele MG, Kolk J, Bets D, Verburg J, Donker AJM, Stehouwer CDA. Long Term Treatment with Metformin in Patients with Type 2 Diabetes and Risk of Vitamin B12 Deficiency: Randomised Placebo Controlled Trial. BMJ. 2010; 340:1-7.

[116] Jeetendra S and Tushar B. Metformin Use and Vitamin B12 Deficiency in Patients with Type 2 Diabetes Mellitus. MVP Journal of Medical Sciences. 2016; 3(1):67-70

[117] Kibirige D and Mwebaze R. Vitamin B12 Deficiency among Patients with Diabetes Mellitus: Is Routine Supplementation Justified? Diabetes and Metabolic Disorders. 2013; 12(17):1-6.

[118] Fatima S and Noor S. A Review on Effects of Metformin on Vitamin B12 Status. American Journal of Phytomedicine and Clinical Therapeutics. 2013; 1(8):652-660.

[119] Bodmer M, Meier C, Krahenbuhl S, Jick SS, Meier CR. Metformin, Sulfonylureas, or Other Antidiabetes Drugs and the Risk of Lactic Acidosis or Hypoglycemia. A nested case-control analysis. Diabetes Care. 2008; 31(11):2086-2091. https://doi.org/10.2337/dc08-1171.

[120] Donnelly LA, Dennis JM, Coleman RL, Sattar N, Hattersley AT, Holman RR, Pearson ER. Risk of Anemia with Metformin Use in Type 2 Diabetes: A MASTERMIND Study. Diabetes Care. 2020; dc201104.https://doi.org/10.2337/dc20-1104.

[121] Fujita H, Narita T, Yoshioka N, et al. A case of megaloblastic anemia due to vitamin B12 deficiency precipitated in a totally gastrectomized type II diabetic patient following the introduction of metformin therapy. Endocr J. 2003; 50(4):483-484. doi:10.1507/endocrj.50.483.

[122] Patrick Imfeld, Michael Bodmer, Susan S Jick, Christoph R Meier. Metformin, other antidiabetic drugs, and risk of Alzheimer's disease: a population-based case-control study J Am Geriatr Soc. 2012; 60(5):916-921. doi: 10.1111/j.1532-5415.2012.03916.x.

[123] Moore EM , Mander AG, Ames D, Kotowicz MA, Carne RP, Brodaty H, Woodward M, Boundy K, Ellis KA, Bush AI, Faux NG, Martins R, Szoeke C, Rowe C, Watters DA, AIBL Investigators. Increased risk of cognitive impairment in patients with diabetes is associated with metformin. Diabetes Care. 2013; 36(10):2981-2987. doi: 10.2337/dc13-0229.

[124] Qing ZQ, Shan LW, Zhou L; Zhang, Li HZ, Gui BY, Xia ZR. Metformin therapy and cognitive dysfunction in patients with type 2 diabetes. A meta-analysis and systematic review. Medicine: 2020; 99(10):p e19378. doi: 10.1097/MD.0000000000019378.

[125] Yokoyama H, Ogawa M, Honjo J, et al. Risk factors associated with abnormal cognition in Japanese outpatients with diabetes, hypertension or dyslipidemia. Diabetol Int 2015; 6:268-274.

[126] Zhou Y, Fang R, Liu LH, et al. Clinical characteristics for the relationship between type-2 diabetes mellitus and cognitive impairment: a cross-sectional study. Aging Dis 2015; 6:236-244.

Chapter 5

Interaction Studies of ACE Inhibitors with Antidiabetic Drugs

Safila Naveed and Halima Sadia

Abstract

Angiotensin converting enzyme (ACE)-inhibitors are effective in patients with mild to moderately severe hypertension, collagen vascular and cardiovascular disease. They are also used in the prevention and treatment of myocardial infarction and in the management of cardiac arrhythmias. Patients with cardiovascular diseases are generally on multiple medicines that's why it is imperative to study drug–drug interactions of medicines which are commonly taken together in any given case, as combined administration of different medicines can significantly influence the availability of drugs. In the present study we investigated the "*in vitro*" interactions of ACE inhibitors (enalapril, captopril and lisinopril) with frequently prescribed and co-administered drugs in simulated human body environments. These interactions were monitored by means of UV spectrophotometry and separation technique as RP-HPLC. Prior to start of actual drug interactions, the method of analysis of each drug was established and its various parameters validated for considering its use in testing of drug *in vitro* as well as in human serum. For this purpose, an attempt was made to develop a number of new HPLC methods for determination of ACE inhibitors (enalapril, captopril and lisinopril) and simultaneously with interacting drugs. These methods were optimized, validated and then successfully employed for the quantitation of enalapril, captopril and lisinopril and selected drugs in interactions studies. As a result, new methods for the quantitation of individual as well as multiple drugs were developed. The interacting drugs selected were antidiabetic drugs (metformin, glibenclamide, glimepride and pioglitazone. Interaction consequences revealed that the availability of enalapril was not affected in presence of antidiabetic drugss whereas the availability of captopril and lisinopril were altered in presence of NIDDMs.

Keywords: ACE Inhibitors, Antidiabetics, Interaction studies, HPLC, Method development

1. Introduction

1.1 Angiotensin converting enzyme

Angiotensin Converting Enzyme is an ectoenzyme and a glycoprotein with an appreciate molecular weight of 170,000 Do. Human angiotensin converting enzyme contains 277 aminoacid residues and has two homologous domains, each with a catalytic site and a region for binding Zn^{+2} [1, 2]. The degradation of bradykinin to inactive peptides occurs via action of ACE, thus ACE not only produces a potent vasoconstricton but also inactivates a potent vasodilator [3].

In 1965, Ferreira [4] studied the physiological effects of snake poisoning and discovered a specific component from the venom of the pit viper, *bothrops jararaca*, which inhibits degradation of the peptide bradykinin and potentiate hypotensive action of bradykinin. These factors originally designated as bradykinin potentiating factors (BPFs), were isolated and found to be a family of peptides containing 5–13 amino acid residues. Bakhle [5] reported that these same peptides had an inhibitory activity on ACE of dog lung homogenate and inhibited the enzymatic conversion of angiotensin I to angiotensin II. Hans Brunner and John Laragh [6] administered it to hypertensive patients and showed that it was extremely effective in lowering blood pressure. The structural requirements for substrates of angiotensin converting enzyme to cleave a substrate are found similar to those observed with carboxypeptidase A of bovine pancrease [7, 8]. The substrate specificity and other properties of angiotensin converting enzyme suggested that it was a zinc metallopeptidase, similar in mechanism to carboxypeptidase A, an enzyme whose active site had been well characterized by x-ray crystallography and other methods [9]. In 1970, Ferreira and Greene [10] isolated and characterized the first peptide, a bradykinin-potentiating pentapeptide that they called BPP5a; it also inhibited ACE and transiently lowered blood pressure in animal models. The significance of ACE in the pathogenesis of hypertension was not fully appreciated until 1977's, when Ondetti [11] first isolated and then synthesized the naturally occurring nonpeptide, teprotide. He proposed a hypothetical model of the active site of ACE and used it to predict and design compounds that would occupy the carboxy- terminal binding site of the enzyme [12]. Cushman and Ondetti first created succinyl-L-proline, which showed slight positive activity. Inhibitory activity increased 15 to 20 times when they substituted a methyl group in the 2 position of succinyl group. Finally to enhance the binding capacity of substrate structure and zinc of the enzyme they replaced succinyl COOH with sulf-hydryl, a 2000 times increase in inhibitory potency was achieved. ACE inhibitors entered the antihypertensive drug market during the 1980. Manolio [13] explored new types of drugs in preventing cardiovascular mortality. Captopril, a specific potent inhibitor of ACE, showed excellent anti-hypertensive properties in clinical trials and had a major impact on the treatment of cardiovascular disease [14].

1.1.1 Chemistry

The most thoroughly studied of the peptide inhibitors of converting enzyme is the nonapeptide known as teprotide, having the structure, Pyoglu-Tro-Arg-Pro-Glnlle-Pro-Pro.Teprotide acts as a competitive inhibitor of converting enzyme, with an affinity for the enzyme much higher than that of angiotensin I. It is not itself a substrate for the enzyme. Although converting enzyme will cleave many different C-terminal dipeptide residues, it will not cleave peptides with proline in the penultimate position. As noted, the penultimate proline in angiotensin II, indeed, is responsible for its refractoriness to further cleavage by converting enzyme. Moreover, the presence of Pyro Glu at the N-terminus renders teprotide refractory to amino peptidases; this confers further stability and effectiveness in vivo. Nevertheless, teprotide has a relatively short duration of action and must be given parentally to be effective [11]. The optimum pH of angiotensin converting enzyme was found to vary with the substrate employed and to be influenced by the presence or absence of chloride ion. With longer peptide substrates such as angiotensin I or bradykinin in the presence of chloride ion, the optimal pH for hydrolytic action of the converting enzyme was about 7.5; with tripeptide substrates such as Z-Phe-His-Leu, Hip-His-Leu, or Hip-Gly-Gly, it was about pH 8.5 [15, 16]. Studies of the hydrolysis of synthetic substrate of ACE [17, 18] and hippuryl di and tripeptides [19] shows that enzyme tolerate changes at antepenultimate position of a peptide substrate especially aromatic amino acids such as phenylalanine which contributes greatly to the overall affinity for the enzyme. A tripeptide with an acylated terminal amino group is the simplest peptide cleaved by the enzyme. However, the tripeptide Z-Phe-His-Leu, analogous to the terminal tripeptide sequence of angiotensin I, binds to the active site of angiotensin converting enzyme as well as the intact decapeptide. Peptides such as angiotensin II with a penultimate proline residue [20]. The orally effective ACE-inhibitor was developed by a rational approach that involved analysis of the inhibitory action of teprotide, inferences about the action of converting enzyme on its substrates, and analogy with carboxy peptidase A, which was known to be inhibited by d-benzylsuccinic acid. Ondetti and Cushman urged that inhibition of converting enzyme might be produced by succinyl amino acids that corresponded in length to the dipeptide cleaved by converting enzyme. This proved to be true and led ultimately to the synthesis of a series of carboxy or mercapto alkanoyl derivatives that acted as competitive inhibitors of the enzyme [21].

1.1.2 Mechanism of action

These drugs block the angiotensin converting enzyme that cleaves the terminal two peptides from angiotensin I (decapeptide) to form the potent vasoconstrictor angiotensin II (octapeptide) [22, 23] and lower the BP by reducing peripheral vascular resistance without reflexly increasing cardiac out put rate, and contractility [22]. They also inhibit the rate of bradykinin inactivation thus resulting in vasodilation, they also decrease the secretion of aldisterone resulting in decrease of sodium and water retention.

1.1.3 Pharmacokinetics

ACE-inhibitors are given by mouth, the oral bioavailability of this class of drugs ranges from 13–95% [24, 25]. Most of the ACE inhibitors are administered as prodrugs that remain inactive until esterified in the liver [26]. Fosinoprilate is excreted via biliary duct, elimination of the diacid is polyphasic and there is a prolong terminal elimination phase, which is considered to represent binding to ACE at saturate binding site. This bond fraction does not contribute to accumulation of drug following multiple doses [27, 28].

1.1.4 Therapeutic use

ACE-inhibitors are effective in patients with mild to moderately severe hypertension, with normal or low plasma renin activity, with collagen vascular disease, with cardiovascular and in anephric disease [29–36]. They cause a reduction in left ventricular hypertrophy, and in plasma fibrinogen level [37, 38]. They are also used in the prevention and treatment of myocardial infarction [39, 40], and in the management of cardiac arrhythmias [41, 42]. They can decrease the progression of atherosclerosis [43], microalbuminuria [44] and diabetic retinopathy [45–47] and produce beneficial effect in Bartter's syndrome [48].

1.1.5 Adverse effects

Pronounced hypertension may occur at the start of therapy with ACE-inhibitors particularly in patients with heart failure, and in sodium or volume depletion patients [49–51]. They cause hyperkalemia in patients with renal insufficiency or in patients taking k + −sparing diuretic, k + −supplement, beta blockers or NSAID's [23, 52] and produce cough in hypertensive patient [53, 54]. Altered liver function, cholestatic jaundice, hepatitis, hepatotoxicity [55] and aplastic anemia [56] have also been reported. They can produce a complex and contradictory effect on kidney and induce renal insufficiency in patients having bilateral renal artery stenosis, heart failure or diarrhea [57–61]. Angioedema is a rare but potentially life-threatening side effect of ACE inhibitors [62–68] can cause a number of fetal anomalies [69, 70]. Scalded mouth syndrome [71] and drug induced pulmonary-infiltration with eosinophilia syndrome (PIE-syndrome) is a rare complication [72]. With use of ACE inhibitors, anaphylactoid reactions are also reported [73, 74].

1.1.6 Contraindications

Experimental and clinical data conclude that use of ACE inhibitors should be avoided in all trimester of pregnancy [75, 76]. Patients with peripheral vascular disease are at high risk of renal failure with this therapy [77] also contraindicated in known hypersensitivity to any ACE inhibitors [78].

1.1.7 Overdosage

There have been reports of over dosages with captopril and enalepril [79–81], the main effect is hypotension [82, 83] which usually responds to supportive treatment and volume expansion, pressor agents are rarely required. Infusion of angiotensin amide may be considered if hypotension persists [84, 85].

1.1.8 Drug interactions

Hypotensive effect of ACE inhibitors decreased when given in combination with non-steroidal anti-inflammatory drugs [86] but this effect is enhanced with calcium-channel blockers [87] and beta-blockers [88]. Granulocytopenia occurs after combine therapy of ACE inhibitors and interferones [89], the nitritoid reaction occurs with concomitant use of gold salt and ACE inhibitors [90]. Cytokines antagonize the hypotensive effect of ACE inhibitors [91], severe hypokalaemia occurs with potassium depleting diuretics [92] and potassium-sparing diuretics produced hyperkalaemia [93–95]. ACE inhibitors could increase potassium levels in the body [96, 97]. Alpha-blockers enhance hypotensive effect of ACE inhibitors [98]. Iron supplementation successfully decreases cough induced by ACE-inhibitors [99] and can interfere with the absorption of ACE inhibitors [100]. Hypoglycemic effect is enhanced with antidiabetics and insulin [101, 102]. Azathioprine and ACE inhibitors combination is associated with anemia [103]. Marked hypotension occurs in patients receiving general anesthetics and ACE inhibitors [104]. The risk of bone marrow depression is increased in patients taking concomitant therapy of ACE-inhibitors and immunosuppressive agents [76]. **Table 1** shows some example of ACE Inhibitors.

1.2 Antidiabetic drugs

Type II or non insulin dependent diabetes mellitus (NIDDM) formerly known as maturity-onset or adult-onset diabetes. Approximately 95% of patients are being affected by the type II form [105, 106]. NIDDM are being increasingly diagnosed as its importance as a risk factor for the development of cardiovascular disease and many drugs has been known to interfere with glucose control. The greatest effect was seen with propranolol and the least with cardioselective and less lipophilic beta-blockers, nifedipine has been associated with deterioration in glucose control but verapamil has been found to have a beneficial effect on glucose control. Antihypertensive drug clonidine has not been shown to result in deterioration in glucose control when used in NIDDM. Long term therapy with the more specific agonist guanfacine was reported to have a beneficial effect on glucose tolerance [107]. **Table 2** shows, examples of antidiabetic drugs.

Drugs	Nomenclature	Structure
Enalapril	(S)-1-[N-[1-(ethoxycarbonyl)-3-phenyl propyl]-L-alanyl]-L-proline, (Z)-2-butenedioate salt	
Captopri1	1-(3-mercapto-2-dmethyl-1-oxopropyl)-1-proline (S,S)	
Lisinopri1	((S)-1-[N2-(1-carboxy-3-phenylpropyl)-1-lysyl]-1-proline dehydrate	

Table 1.
Examples of ACE inhibitors.

Drags	Nomenclature	Structure
Pioglitizone	(±)-5-[[4-[2-(methyl-2-pyridinylamino) ethoxy]phenyl]methyl]-2,4-thiazolidinedione, (Z)-2-butenedioate(1:1)	
Glibenclamide	1-[[4-[2-[(5-chloro-2-ethoxybenzoyl)amino]ethyl]phenyl]sulphonyl]-3-cyclohexylurea, $C_{23}H_{28}ClN_3O_5S$	
Metformin	N,N-dimethyl-imido-di-carbonimidic diamide hydrochloride	
Glimepride	[[p-[2-(3-ethyl-4-methyl-2-oxo-3-pyyroline-1-oxamide)ethyl]phenyl] sulfonyl]-3-(trans-4-methylcyclohexyl) urea,	

Table 2.
Examples of anti-diabetic.

2. Experimental

2.1 Materials

Raw materials used were of pharmaceutical purity and were obtained from different Pharmaceutical Companies (**Table 3**). Tablets were purchased from local

Class	Drugs	Brands	Potency (mg)	Pharmaceutical industry
ACE inhibitors	Enalapril	Renitec	10	MSD
	Captopril	Capoten	25	Bristol Meyers Pvt. Ltd
	Lisinopril	Lisinopril	5	Atco Laboratories Ltd
Antidiabetic	Metformin	Neodipar	250	Sanofi Aventis (Pakistan) Ltd
	Glimepride	Amaryl	2	Sanofi Aventis (Pakistan) Ltd
	Pioglitazone	Poze	45	Ali Goliar Pharmaceuticals (Pvt
	Glibenclamide	Diazet	5	Safe Pharmaceutical (Pvt) Ltd

Table 3.
Drugs, brands and manufacturers.

pharmacy and each product was labeled and expiry date not earlier than two years, at the time of these studies were noted.

2.1.1 Reagents

Analytical grade reagents were used during the whole experimental procedures. Methanol and acetonitrile were of (HPLC grade) (TEDIA®, USA). Other reagents include hydrochloric acid, sodium hydroxide, sodium chloride, potassium dihydrogen orthophosphate, disodium hydrogen orthophosphate, ammonium chloride, 10% NH_3 solution, phosphoric acid 85% (Merk, Germany). Organic solvents used were methanol, ethanol, ethyl acetate, chloroform, acetronitrile, triethylamine and DMSO (Merck Grade).

2.1.2 Equipments

UV visible spectrophotometer (Model 1601, Shimadzu, Japan) with 10-mm path length connected to a P-IV computer loaded with Shimadzu UVPC version 3.9 software was used in these studies. Deionizer, Stedec CSW-300 used for deionization of water. The dissolution equipment was the B.P. 2009 standards. Chromatographic studies were carried out by using two Shimadzu HPLC systems, one equipped with LC-10 AT VP pump, SPD-10 A VP UV–*vis* detector and other HPLC system was equipped with LC-20AT and SPD-20A UV/VIS detector utilizing Hypersil, ODS, C18 (150 × 4.6 mm, 5micron) and Purospher® STAR RP-18 column. Chromatographic data were recorded using a CBM-102 Shimadzu. Shimadzu Class-GC 10 software (version 2) for data acquisition and mathematical calculations.

IR studies were carried out by FTIR Prestige-21 spectrophotometer Shimadzu. Spectral treatment was performed using Shimadzu IRsolution 1.2 software. The H^1-NMR spectra were recorded on a Bruker AMX 500 MHz spectrometer using TMS as an internal standard. Melting points were recorded by Gallenkamp melting point apparatus.

2.2 Methods

2.2.1 Preparation of simulated gastric juice and buffers

0.1 N hydrochloric acid was prepared by diluting 9 mL hydrochloric acid of analytical grade (11 N) in a liter volumetric flask and the volume was made up to the mark with de-ionized water. Chloride buffer of pH 4 was prepared by dissolving

3.725 g of potassium chloride in deionized water in one liter and 0.1 N HCl was used for pH adjustment. For preparation of phosphate buffer of pH 7.4, 0.6 gm of potassium dihydrogen orthophosphate, 6.4 g of disodium hydrogen orthophosphate and 5.85 g of sodium chloride were dissolved in sufficient deionized water to produce 1000 mL and the pH adjusted. For preparation of ammonia buffer of pH 9, 4.98 g of ammonium chloride was dissolved in 1000 mL of deionized water and pH adjusted with 10% ammonia.

2.2.2 Construction of the calibration curve of drugs

The above prepared working standard solutions of all drugs were scanned in the region 200–700 nm against the reagent blank and absorbance maxima was recorded as shown in **Table 4**. Calibration curves were constructed between concentration and absorbance. Epsilon values and linear coefficients were calculated in each case at all above described pH values. Beer Lambert's law was obeyed at all concentrations and pH.

2.2.3 Monitoring of drug interactions of enalapril, captopril and lisinopril by high performance liquid chromatography

HPLC methods for simultaneous determination of enalapril, captopril and lisinopril with NSAIDs, H_2-receptor antagonist, statins, antidiabetic drugs, metals and antacids in raw materials, pharmaceutical dosage forms or in human serum are developed and validated according to ICH guidelines. These methods were then applied to drug–drug, drug metals and drug antacid interaction studies.

2.2.4 Chromatographic conditions

The isocratic elution was performed at ambient temperature with two different types of columns. Hypersil, ODS, C18 (150 × 4.6 mm, 5micron) and Purospher® STAR RP-18, for assay of enalapril, captopril and lisinopril and simultaneous determination of these drugs with interacting drugs respectively. The mobile phase, flow rate, wavelength UV detection were varied as cited in **Table 5**. Sample volume of 20 μL was injected in triplicate onto the HPLC column and elute was monitored at different wavelengths.

2.2.5 Preparation of standard solutions

Stock reference standard solutions of all drugs were prepared daily by dissolving appropriate amounts of each drug in mobile phase to yield final concentrations

Class of drugs	Analytes	Wavelength (nm)	Cone.range (m Mole)
ACE inhibitors	Enalapril	203, 206, 207, 208	$1–9 \times 10^{-5}$
	Captopril	203, 204, 206	$5–14 \times 10^{-7}$
	Lisinopril	206	$1–10 \times 10^{-5}$
Antidiabetic drugs	Metformin	205, 223	0.01–0.1
	Glimepride	240	0.01–0.1
	Glibenclamide	231, 238, 246	0.01–0.1
	Pioglitazone	225, 269	0.01–0.1

Table 4.
Absorbance maxima.

Drugs	Mobile phase			pH	Flow rate	Detection
	MeOH	ACN	H$_2$O		mLmin^{-1}	Nm
Enalapril assay	70	—	30	3.5	1	215
Enalapril+Antidiabetic drugs	70		30	2.8	1	230
Captopril	50	—	50	2.9	1	220
Captopril +Antidiabetic drugs	70		30	3	1	230
Lisinopril	80	2.5	17.5	3	1	225
Lisinopril+Antidiabetic drugs	80		20	3	1	225

Table 5.
Chromatographie conditions of HPLC methods.

300 μg mL^{-1}. For the calibration standards, calibrators of each drug were prepared by making serial dilutions from stock solutions. All solutions were filtered through 0.45 μm filter and degassed using sonicator.

2.2.6 Preparation of pharmaceutical dosage form samples

Pharmaceutical formulations of the respective brands, commercially available in Pakistan were evaluated. In each case, groups of twenty tablets were individually weighed and finely powdered in a mortar. Weighed portion of the powder equivalent to the suitable amount of drug (according to the labeled claimed) was transferred into a 100 mL volumetric flask completely dissolved in mobile phase and then diluted with this solvent up to the mark, a portion of this solution was filtered through a disposable 0.45 μm filter and then injected.

2.2.7 Preparation of standard drug plasma solutions

Blood samples were collected from healthy volunteers and then centrifuged at 3000 rpm for 10 minutes and supernatant was stored at −20°C. After thawing, serum was deprotinated by acetonitrile and spiked daily with working solutions to produce desired concentrations of enalapril and interacting drugs. 10 μL volume of each sample was injected and chromatographed under above conditions.

2.3 Method development and optimization

HPLC methods were developed and optimized for certain parameters before method validation. The optimization of the analytical procedure has been carried out by varying the mobile phase composition, flow rate, pH of the mobile phase, diluents of solutions and wavelength of analytes in order to achieve symmetrical peaks with good resolution at reasonable retention time.

2.3.1 Method validation

All validation steps were carried out according to the ICH guidelines such as system suitability, selectivity, specificity, linearity (concentration–detector response relationship), accuracy, precision and sensitivity i.e. detection and quantification limit.

2.3.2 System suitability

System suitability of the method was evaluated by analyzing five replicate analyses of the drug at a specific concentration for repeatability, peaks symmetry

(symmetry factor), theoretical plates of the column, resolution between the peaks of enalapril and other drugs, mass distribution ratio (capacity factor) and relative retention.

2.3.3 Specificity and linearity

The drugs were spiked with pharmaceutical formulations containing different excepients. The linearity of the method was evaluated at different concentrations with different groups. Linear correlation coefficient, intercept and slope values were calculated for statistical analysis.

2.3.4 Accuracy and precision

The accuracy of the method was calculated at three concentration levels (80, 100 and 120%) by spiking known quantities of the drug analytes. Three injections of each solution were injected to HPLC system and % recovery was calculated in each case.

For the precision of the method, six replicates of each level were injected to system on two different non-consecutive days in each case and %RSD was calculated.

2.3.5 Limit of detection and quantification

Detection limit (LOD) of the method was calculated by the formula LOD = 3.3 SD/slope. The quantitation limit (LOQ) is the lowest level of analyte that is accurately measured and it was evaluated as ten times the noise level LOQ =10σ/S; where σ is the standard deviation of the lowest standard concentration and S is the slope of the standard curve.

2.3.6 Robustness

Robustness was performed by making minor changes in the percentage of mobile phase (methanol, water and acetonitrile) wave length, pH and flow rate. Therefore, five repeated samples were injected under small variations of each parameter. When a parameter was changed ±0.2% (in flow rate), ± 0.2% pH and ± 5% wave length from its optimum condition.

2.3.7 Ruggedness

Ruggedness of our method was determined in two different labs. Lab 1 was the Research Institute of Pharmaceutical Sciences, Department of Pharmaceutical Chemistry, Faculty of Pharmacy, University of Karachi while other lab was lab 9, Department of Chemistry, Faculty of Science, University of Karachi. Two different instruments one was LC 10 and LC 20. Two different columns Purospher STAR C_{18} and Hypersil ODS were used.

2.3.8 Interaction studies by HPLC

Enalapril solution was mixed with each solution of interacting drug separately that gave the final concentration of 100μgmL^{-1} for each constituent. These were kept in water bath maintained at 37°C for 3 hours. An aliquot of 5 mL was withdrawn after every 30 minutes intervals, after making appropriate dilutions was filtered through 0.45 μ filter paper and three replicates were injected to HPLC system. The concentration of each drug was determined and % recovery was calculated and the same procedure was applied for captopril and lisinopril.

3. Result and discussion

3.1 Simultaneous quantitation of enalapril and antidiabetic drugs (metformin, glibenclamide and glimepiride)

There are number of HPLC methods reported for the quantitation of metformin using UV detector [108, 109] liquid chromatography–tandem mass spectrometry [110] and from human plasma [111]. Moreover, there are many methods reported for the simultaneous analysis of metformin with other antidiabetics [112, 113]. Likewise, there are methods reported for the analysis of glibenclamide from pharmaceutical formulations [114], human plasma [115, 116] using HPLC. Similarly, there are methods reported for the simultaneous analysis of glibenclamide with other anti-diabetics. However, no method reported in the literature for the simultaneous quantitation of enalapril, metformin, glibenclamide and glimepride.

3.1.1 Method optimization and chromatographic conditions

In the present investigation the best separation of enalapril and antidiabetic drugs was achieved using a Hypersil, ODS, C18 (150 × 4.6 mm, 5micron) column which provides efficient and reproducible separation of the components. Using other type of column under similar experimental condition, the separation lasted about 11 minutes. A mobile phase of methanol: water (70:30 v/v) having pH adjusted with phosphoric acid to 2.8 provided a reproducible, baseline resolved peak. Small changes in pH of the mobile phase had a great influence to the chromatographic behavior of these drugs, higher pH of the mobile phase also results in peak tailing and at a lower pH retention time of antidiabetic drugs and enalapril was delayed. It is obvious from the chromatogram (**Figure 1**) that antidiabetic drugs and enalapril eluted out forming symmetrical peaks and were well separated from each other. The method was found to be rapid as the drugs separated in a very short time i.e. enalapril 3.6 min and metformin, glibenclamide and glimepiride elution time was 2.4, 8.5 and 10.9 min respectively, which is important for routine analysis. The advantages of this method are ease of operation, short analysis time (total run time < 12 minutes), utilization of readily available cost-effective solvents, no matrix interferences, and satisfactory limit of quantification to enable pharmacokinetic studies of enalapril and NIDDMs.

3.1.2 Method validation

The developed method was validated by ICH guidelines [117]. It includes various parameters for example system suitability, selectivity, specificity, linearity, accuracy test, precision, robustness, ruggedness, sensitivity, limit of detection and quantification.

3.1.2.1 System suitability

The HPLC system was equilibrated with the initial mobile phase composition, followed by 6 injections of the same standard to evaluate the system suitability on each day of method validation. Parameters of system suitability are peaks symmetry (symmetry factor), theoretical plates of the column, resolution, mass distribution ratio (capacity factor) and relative retention as summarized in **Table 6**.

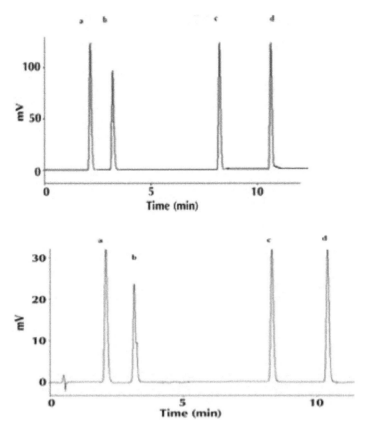

Figure 1.
A representative chromatogram of, and (a) MET (b) ENP (c) GLB (d) GMP in formulation and serum.

Analytes	Retention time (T_R) (mm)	Capacity factors (K')	Theoretical plates (N)	Tailing factor (T)	Resolut ion (R)	Separation factor
ENP	3.6	2.6	3200	1.23	3.3	2.48
MET	2.4	2.9	3250	1.25	3.5	2.56
GLB	8.5	2.89	3256	1.26	3.6	2.59
GMP	10.9	2.69	3246	1.28	3.9	2.69

Table 6.
System suitability parameters.

3.1.2.2 Linearity

Linearity is generally reported as the variance of the slope of the regression line. Linearity was tested with known concentrations of ENP, MET, GLB and GMP i.e. 2.5, 5, 10, 25, 50 and 100 μgmL^{-1} respectively. Injected concentrations versus area were plotted and the correlation coefficients were calculated which are shown in **Table 7**.

Drugs	Conc. μgmL^{-1}	Regression Equation	r^2	LOD	LOQ
				μgmL^{-1}	
ENP	2.5–100	y = 2489.4x + 255.5	0.9996	1.53	4.6
MET	2.5–100	y = 10406x + 24139	0.9993	0.317	0.96
GLB	2.5–100	y = 14651x + 33832	0.9998	0.19	0.58
GMP	2.5–100	y = 15438x + 39969	0.9996	0.1	0.32

Table 7.
Regresssion statistics LOD and LOQ.

3.1.2.3 Accuracy

Method accuracy was evaluated as the percentage of recovery by estimation of all investigated analytes in presence of various commonly used tablets' excepients at three levels of concentrations that were 80, 100 and 120%. Each sample was injected five times and accuracy was determined in range of 98.6–102.3% (**Table 8**). No significant difference observed between amounts added and recovered without serum and with serum. Thus, used excepients did not interfere with active present in tablets.

3.1.2.4 Precision

Precision was evaluated by carrying out six independent sample preparation of a single lot of formulation. The sample solution was prepared in the same manner as described in sample preparation. Percentage relative standard deviation (%RSD) was found to be less than 2% for within a day and day to day variations, which proves that method is precise. Results are shown in **Table 9**.

3.1.2.5 Sensitivity

The limit of quantitation (LOQ) of the method as signal/noise of ENP, MET, GLB and GMP were found to be 4.6, 0.96, 0.58 and 0.32 μgmL^{-1} respectively.

Analytes	Assay (spiking method)			Assay in serum	
	Conc. μgmL-1	%RSD	% Rec	%RSD	%Rec
ENP	8	0.011	101	0.9	100.3
	10	0.326	100.3	0.23	101.23
	12	0.001	100	0.8	102
MET	8	0.007	100.6	0.96	101
	10	0.002	100.9	0.56	99.98
	12	0.001	100.5	0.89	101.3
GLB	8	0.008	99.7	0.69	99.69
	10	0.002	99.9	0.69	101.6
	12	0.001	100	1.03	102.3
GMP	8	0.008	99.7	0.89	101.3
	10	0.002	100.2	0.36	98.36
	12	0.001	100.1	1.02	99.89

Table 8.
Accuracy of ENP and NIDDM drugs.

Drugs	Conc. injected μgmL^{-1}	Inter-day		Intra-day	
		%RSD	%Rec	%RSD	%Rec
ENP	2.5	0.4	97.44	0.96	100.9
	5	0.3	100.5	0.63	101.1
	10	0.2	99.87	0.65	99.49
	25	0.11	99.2	0.63	101.2
	50	0.56	100.8	0.62	98.94
	100	0.36	99.92	0.62	101.1
MET	2.5	0.35	97.4	0.63	100.9
	5	0.36	102	0.89	101.1
	10	0.9	99.5	0.5	100.9
	25	0.56	101	0.63	100.5
	50	0.25	101	0.36	99.45
	100	1	100	0.63	100.6
GLB	2.5	1.2	97.6	0.07	100
	5	1.3	100.8	1.56	101
	10	1.02	100	0.56	101
	25	1.03	102	0.57	101
	50	1.03	100.2	0.63	99.1
	100	1.05	101.8	0.69	99.6
GMP	2.5	0.69	99.2	0.36	98.85
	5	0.65	102	1.02	99.5
	10	0.68	100	0.9	100.55
	25	1.65	102	0.9	101.19
	50	0.07	100.1	1.2	98.14
	100	0.36	101.6	0.65	99.58

Table 9.
Inter day and intraday precision of ENP and NIDDM drugs.

Similarly a signal/noise of 3, a LOD of ENP, MET, GLB and GMP were determined to be 1.53, 0.317, 0.19, and 0.1 μgmL^{-1} respectively.

3.1.2.6 Ruggedness

The ruggedness of this method was calculated in two different labs with two different instruments. The method did not show any notable deviations in results from acceptable limits.

3.1.2.7 Robustness of method

To evaluate the robustness of the developed RP-HPLC method, small deliberate variations in the optimized method parameters were done. The effect of change in flow rate, pH and mobile phase ratio on the retention time and tailing factor were studied. The method was found to be unaffected by small changes like ±0.1 change in pH, ± 0.1 change in flow rate and ± 1 change in mobile phase.

3.2 Simultaneous determination of captopril and antidiabetic drugs (metformin, pioglitazone and glibenclamide)

The aim of the present study was to establish an efficient, reliable, accurate, precise and sensitive method for the separation and quantitative determination of both drugs simultaneously. These drugs belonged to different classes that could be co-administrated in a number of cases. Simultaneous determination of these drugs is desirable as this would allow more efficient generation of clinical data and could be performed at more modest cost than separate assays. We have developed the method for the simultaneous determination of captopril, metformin, pioglitazone and glibenclamide. The method has been validated according to ICH guidelines and was found to be reproducible. Further, this validated method was used to study the possible *in vitro* interactions of captopril with (metformin, pioglitazone and glibenclamide). Several problems were resolved in the simultaneous determination of compounds investigated.

3.2.1 Method optimization and chromatographic conditions

To optimize the operating conditions for isocratic RP-LC detection of all analytes, a number of parameters such as the mobile phase composition, pH and the flow rate were varied. Various ratios (50:50, 60:40, 70:30 v/v) of methanol: water were tested as starting solvent for system suitability study. The variation in the mobile phase leads to considerable changes in the chromatographic parameters, like peak symmetry, capacity factor and retention time. The pH effect showed that optimized conditions are reached when the pH value is 2.8, producing well resolved and sharp peaks for all drugs assayed. However, the ratio of (70:30 v/v) methanol: water pH adjusted to 2.8 with phosphoric acid as mobile phase (filtered through a 0.45 micron filter), a flow rate of 1.0 mLmin^{-1} using wavelength 230 nm was chosen as optimal condition. Retention time for captopril was found to be 3.3 minute, metformin, pioglitazone and glibenclamide 2.4, 2.8, 7.2 minutes respectively (**Figure 2**).

3.2.2 Method validation

The developed method was validated by ICH guidelines [5]. It includes various parameters for example system suitability, selectivity, specificity, linearity, accuracy test, precision, robustness, ruggedness, sensitivity, limit of detection and quantification (**Table 10**).

3.2.2.1 Linearity

Linearity was studied by preparing standard solutions at different concentration levels. The linearity range for CAP and antidiabetics was found to be 2.5–100 µgmL^{-1} and 0.625–25 µgmL^{-1}, respectively, regression equations for CAP and antidiabetics are given in **Table 11**.

3.2.2.2 Accuracy

Method accuracy was evaluated as the percentage of recovery by estimation of all investigated analytes in presence of various commonly used tablets' excepients at three levels of concentrations that were 80, 100 and 120%. Each sample was injected five times and accuracy was determined in range of 98.45–102.2%. No significant difference was observed between amounts added and recovered without serum and with serum (**Table 12**).

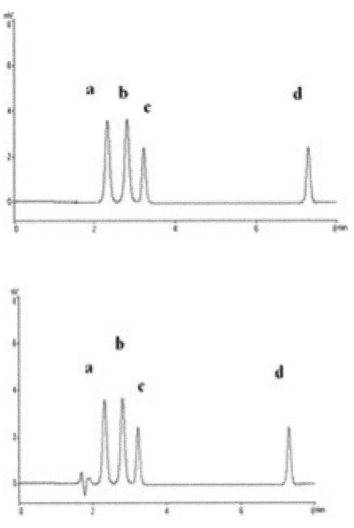

Figure 2.
A representative chromatogram of (a) metformin (b) pioglitazone (c) captopril and (d) glibenclamide in formulation.

3.2.2.3 Precision

Precision was evaluated by carrying out six independent sample preparations of a single lot of formulation. The sample solution was prepared in the same manner as described in sample preparation. Percentage relative standard deviation (%RSD) was found to be less than 2% for within a day and day to day variations, which proves that method is precise (**Table 13**).

3.2.2.4 Sensitivity

The limit of quantitation (LOQ) of the method as signal/noise of CAP, MET, PGL and GLB were found to be 2.3, 1.5, 2.3and 2.3 µgmL^{-1} respectively. Similarly a signal/noise of 3, a LOD of CAP, MET, PGL and GLB were determined to be 0.7, 0.4, 0.7, and 0.7 µgmL^{-1}, respectively.

Analytes	Retention time (T_R) (min)	Capacity factors (K')	Theoretical plates (N)	Tailing factor (T)	Resolution (R)	Separation factor
CAP	3.3	2.13	3200	1.23	3.4	2.48
MET	2.4	2.25	3250	1.25	3.5	2.36
PGL	2.8	2.36	3250	1.36	3.6	2.59
GLB	7.2	2.36	3246	1.69	3.3	2.56

Table 10.
System suitability parameters.

Drugs	Conc. μgmL^{-1}	Regression equation	r^2	LOD	LOQ
				μgmL^{-1}	
CAP	2.5–100	A = 2501.7x + 3073.7	0.9995	0.7	2.3
MET	2.5–100	A = 3841.3x + 4744.2	0.9998	0.4	1.5
PIO	2.5–100	A = 2419.8x + 2988.8	0.9995	0.7	2.3
GLB	2.5–100	A = 2419.8x + 2988.8	0.9995	0.7	2.3

Table 11.
Regression characteristics.

Analyte	Assay (spiking method)			Assay in serum	
	Conc. μgmL^{-1}	%RSD	% Rec	%RSD	%Rec
CAP	8	0.01	99.98	0.002	102
	10	0.33	100.04	0.02	101
	12	0.36	99.97	0.03	101
MET	8	0.01	100	0.002	101
	10	0	100.02	0.002	101.3
	12	0.3	99.98	0.02	100.3
PGL	8	0.22	99.3	0.03	100.2
	10	0.4	99.98	0.036	100.6
	12	99.73	79.79	0.3	101.3
GLB	8	0.01	99.73	0.06	101.3
	10	0.3	100.24	0.05	101.6
	12	0.5	100.06	0.06	102.0

Table 12.
Accuracy of captopril and antidiabetic drugs.

3.2.2.5 Ruggedness

Ruggedness of this method was evaluated in two different labs with two different instruments. The method did not show any notable deviations in results from acceptable limits.

Drugs	Conc. injected µgmL^{-1}	Inter-day		Intra-day	
		%RSD	%Rec	%RSD	%Rec
CAP	2.5	0.0073	101.11	0.073	101.11
	5	0.0109	102.36	0.009	102.36
	10	0.3261	100	0.361	100.02
	25	0.0009	100	0.09	100.03
	50	0.0005	99.826	0.005	99.26
	100	0.0002	99.998	0.002	99.98
MET	1.25	0.0047	99.997	0.047	99.9
	2.5	0.0071	99.988	0.071	99.88
	5	0.0024	100.12	0.024	100.1
	10	0.0006	99.983	0.006	99.93
	25	0.0006	99.968	0.006	99.98
	50	0.0003	99.991	0	99.91
PGL	1.25	0.0075	98.72	0.007	98.72
	2.5	0.0075	99.98	0.075	99.98
	5	0.0019	99.73	0.019	99.73
	10	0.0012	99.97	0.012	99.87
	25	0.0005	99.97	0.005	99.87
	50	0.0003	100.02	0.003	100.1
GLB	1.25	0.008	100.02	0.08	100.2
	2.5	0.008	99.783	0.008	99.7
	5	0.002	99.983	0.002	99.9
	10	0.001	99.972	0.001	99.9
	25	5.00E-04	99.996	5.00E-04	99.9
	50	3.00E-04	99.997	3.00E-04	99.9

Table 13.
Inter day and intraday precision of captopril and NIDDM drugs.

3.2.2.6 Robustness of method

To evaluate the robustness of the developed RP-HPLC method, small deliberate variations in the optimized method parameters were done. The effect of change in flow rate, pH and mobile phase ratio on the retention time and tailing factor were studied. The method was found to be unaffected by small changes like ±0.1 change in pH, ± 0.1 change in flow rate and ± 1 change in mobile phase.

3.3 Simultaneous determinations of lisinopril, pioglitazone, glibenclamide and glimepiride

There is no method reported for the simultaneous determination of LSP and antidiabetic drugs using HPLC however there are methods for the determination of lisinopril [118, 119], similarly, there are methods reported for the simultaneous analysis of anti-diabetics. An isocratic reversed phase high-performance liquid chromatographic (RP-HPLC) method has been developed for the simultaneous determination of lisinopril and antidiabetic drugs pioglitazone, glibenclamide and glimepride in bulk, dosage formulations and human serum and used for interaction studies.

3.3.1 Method optimization and chromatographic conditions

To develop a precise, accurate and suitable RP- HPLC method for the simultaneous estimation of LSP with antidiabetic drugs, different mobile phases were tried and the proposed chromatographic conditions were found to be appropriate for the quantitative determination. The short analysis time (<8 min) also enables its application in routine and quality-control analysis of finished products. pH of mobile phase containing methanol: water (80:20),was adjusted to 2.9 with phosphoric acid.The mobile phase was filtered on a 0.45 micron filter and then sonicated for 10 min. The flow rate was set to 1.0 mLmin^{-1}. The retention time for LSP was found to be 2.0 minute pioglitazone 2.6 minute, for glibenclamide was 5.3 minute and glimepride 6.1 minute.

3.3.2 Method validation

The developed method was validated by ICH guidelines, it includes system suitability, selectivity, specificity, linearity, accuracy test, precision, robustness, ruggedness, sensitivity, limit of detection and quantification.

3.3.2.1 System suitability

The HPLC system was equilibrated initially with the mobile phase, followed by 6 injections of the same standard to evaluate the system suitability on each day of method validation. Parameters of system suitability are peaks symmetry (symmetry factor), theoretical plates of The column, resolution, mass distribution ratio (capacity factor) and relative retention as summarized in **Table 14**.

3.3.2.2 Linearity

Linearity was studied by preparing standard solutions at different concentration levels. The linearity range for LSP, PGL, GLB and GMP was found to be 2.5–100 µgmL^{-1}. The regression equation for LSP and antidiabetic drugs were given in **Table 15**.

3.3.2.3 Accuracy

The accuracy of the method was evaluated as the percent recovery by estimation of all investigated analytes in presence of various commonly used tablets' excepients at three levels of concentrations that were 80, 100 and 120%. Each sample was injected five times and accuracy was determined in range of 98.45–102.2%. No significant difference observed between amounts added and recovered without serum and with serum (**Table 16**). Thus, used excepients did not interfere with active present in tablets (**Figure 3**).

3.3.2.4 Ruggedness

Ruggedness of the method was calculated in two different labs with two different instruments. The method did not show any notable deviations from acceptable limits.

Analytes	Retention time (T_R) (min)	Capacity factors (K)	Theoretical plates (N)	Tailing factor (T)	Resolution (R)	Separation factor
LSP	2	2.13	3200	1.23	3.4	2.3
PGL	2.6	2.25	3250	1.25	3.2	2
GLB	5.3	2.36	3250	1.23	3.6	2.59
GMP	6.1	2.5	3246	1.25	3.3	2.1

Table 14.
System suitability parameters.

Drugs	Conc. μgmL^{-1}	Regression equations	r^2	LOD	LOQ
				μgmL^{-1}	
LSP	2.5–100	y = 1788.4x + 2214	0.9995	0.53	1.6
PGL	2.5–100	y = 2419.8x + 2988.8	0.9995	0.07	0.23
GLB	2.5–100	y = 17605x + 14118	0.9992	0.09	0.29
GMP	2.5–100	y = 15254x + 21932	0.9992	0.04	0.12

Table 15.
Regression statistics LOD and LOQ.

Analyte	Assay (spiking method)			Assay in serum	
	Conc. μgmL^{-1}	%RSD	% Rec	%RSD	%Rec
LSP	8	0.23	100	36	102
	10	0.326	100.23	54	100.36
	12	0.23	99.9	0.96	100.69
PGL	8	0.28	100	1.2	99.98
	10	0.36	100	1.3	101.3
	12	0.001	100	1.02	101.3
GLB	8	0.96	99.7	1.03	100.2
	10	0.96	99.9	1.05	102.02
	12	0.26	101	1.06	101.3
GMP	8	0.56	99.7	1.02	101.3
	10	0.32	100.2	0.69	100.69
	12	0.69	100.2	0.96	102.03

Table 16.
Accuracy of LSP and NIDDM drugs.

3.3.2.5 Precision

Precision was evaluated by carrying out six independent sample preparation of a single lot of formulation. The sample solution was prepared in the same manner as described earlier. Relative standard deviation was found to be less than 2% for within a day and day to day variations, which proves that method is precise (**Table 17**).

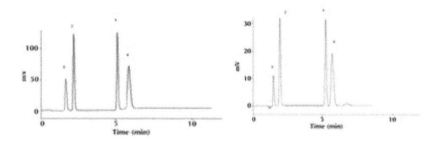

Figure 3.
A representative chromatogram of (1) lisinopril (2) pioglitazone (3) glibenclamide and (4) glimepride in formulation and serum.

Drugs	Conc. injected	Inter-day		Intra-day	
	µgmL⁻¹	%RSD	%Rec	%RSD	%Rec
LSP	2.5	0.3	100.9	1.3	100.8
	5	0.36	101.1	1.3	101
	10	0.6	99.49	1.6	100.4
	25	0.9	101.2	0.6	101.2
	50	0.6	99.32	1.5	100
	100	0.26	100.2	1.08	100
PGL	2.5	1.3	100.9	1.03	99.9
	5	1.3	101.1	1.02	100.2
	10	1.2	100.9	1.32	100.2
	25	0.3	100.5	1.02	101.2
	50	0.65	99.45	0.3	98.9
	100	0.36	100.6	0.96	101.2
GLB	2.5	1.3	100.0	1.02	100
	5	1.2	101.0	0.63	100
	10	1.0.	101.0	1.03	100
	25	1.02	100.0	1.02	100
	50	1.23	99.1	1.023	100
	100	1.23	99.6	1.03	99.6
GMP	2.5	1.6	98.85	1.02	100.2
	5	0.3	99.5	1.03	100.02
	10	1.0	100.5	0.36	100.55
	25	0.02	101.1	0.36	100.23
	50	10.2	98.1	0.23	100.3
	100	1.02	99.5	0.65	99.89

Table 17.
Inter day and intraday precision of LSP and N1DDMdrugs.

3.3.2.6 Sensitivity

Limits of quantitation of the method as signal/noise of 10, for lisinopril, pioglitazone, glibenclamide and glimepride were found to be 1.6, 0.23, 0.29 and 0.12 µgmL⁻¹respectively. Similarly a signal/noise of 3, LOD of lisinopril, pioglitazone glibenclamide and glimepiride were determined to be 0.53, 0.07, 0.09 and 0.04 µgmL⁻¹.

3.3.2.7 Robustness of method

To evaluate the robustness of the developed RP-HPLC method, small deliberate variations in the optimized method parameters were done. The effect of change in flow rate, pH and mobile phase ratio on the retention time and tailing factor were studied. The method was found to be unaffected by small changes like ±0.1 change in pH, ± 0.1 change in flow rate and ± 1 change in mobile phase.

3.4 Interaction of ACE inhibitors with antidiabetic drugs

Hypertension in diabetics represents an important health problem as the combination of these diseases is common, carries significant morbidity and mortality and is frequently difficult to treat. The prevalence of hypertension in diabetic people is probably 1.5–2 times higher than in the general population [118]. Reduction of cardiovascular risk is therefore a high priority in the management of diabetes. Micro albuminuria is an important predictor of cardiovascular events and forms one of the components of insulin resistance/metabolic syndrome, which confers a particularly high risk of cardiovascular death [119]. Diverse classes of antihypertensive prescription may be used for blood pressure manage in diabetes among these angiotensin-II type 1 receptor blockers (ARBs), calcium channel blockers, thiazide diuretics and ACE inhibitors are common [120]. Cheung demonstrated that the calcium antagonists have been extensively used in hypertensive patients with diabetes [121]. Use of Verapamil a calcium channel blocker significantly reduced the risk of developing diabetes [122]. Similarly diabetic patients often take anti-hypertensive medications and coadministered with antidiabetic drugs [123]. Treatment of patients with hypertension and diabetes with ARBs improved both macrovascular and microvascular alterations [124].

Diverse classes of antihypertensive prescription may be used for blood pressure manage in diabetes among these calcium channel blockers, angiotensin-II type 1 receptor blockers (ARBs), thiazide diuretics and ACE inhibitors are common. Cheung demonstrated that calcium antagonists have been extensively used in hypertensive patients with diabetes. Collective pharmacological treatment generally entails in management of type 2 diabetes mellitus to attain satisfactory glucose manage and dealing of concomitant pathologies, drug–drug interactions must be cautiously considered with antihyperglycaemic drugs [125]. Mitra [126] conducted a study to examine the interaction of diabecon (D-400), a herbomineral anti-diabetic the most important purpose of this cram was to assess the *"in vitro"* drug interaction of enalapril, captopril and lisinopril with commonly prescribed antidiabetic drugs (metformin, pioglitazone glimepride and glibenclamide) by utilizing HPLC.

3.4.1 Interaction of enalapril with antidiabetic drugs by HPLC

In vitro interactions of enalapril in the presence of antidiabetic drugs (metformin, glibenclamide and glimepride) were carried out in 1:1 at 37°C and method for simultaneous determination of both interacting drugs was also developed as described in former sections. Results of these interactions are summarized in **Table 18** and plotted in **Figure 4**. The % availability of enalapril and metformin was found to be between 98 and 106% indicating no reaction between drugs. These results clearly indicated that enalapril could be safely co administered with metformin. The two drugs did not inhibit or disturb the absorption of each other. Similar behavior was observed with glibenclamide and glimepride, the availability of enalapril was found to be between 102 and 103% with glibenclamide and

Time	ENP	MET	ENP	GLB	ENP	GMP
0	99.89	100.01	100.34	100.34	102	99.99
30	99.65	99.02	99.54	99.54	101.3	100
60	100.23	95.31	98.12	98.99	102.3	101
90	101.61	105.56	99.69	99.69	102.3	102.3
120	100.2	98.3	98.46	98.46	101.2	102
150	101.98	98.88	100.3	100.63	102.3	103
180	106.46	99.99	100.36	100.36	102.3	104.3

Table 18.
% availability of enalapril and antidiabetic drugs by HPLC.

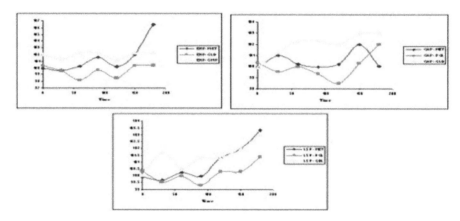

Figure 4.
% Availability of a inhibitors and antidiabetic drugs by HPLC.

glimepride and the availability of glibenclamide and glimepride remained almost unchanged. No remarkable change in area under curve and drift in retention time were observed. However, the results showed that no interaction occurred as there % recovery remained almost unchanged.

3.4.2 Interaction of captopril with antidiabetic drugs by HPLC

In this study drugs were analyzed by measuring the area under curve (AUC), % recovery and considerable drift in retention time. Captopril and metformin did not affect the availabilities of each other i.e. 101% and 103% was observed respectively up to 30 minutes and at the end of experiment both were available up to 100% and 105% respectively. Similar effect was observed in presence of pioglitazone i.e. 102% of captopril, while 104% of pioglitazone was available at the end. In presence of glibenclamide, the %availability of captopril and glibenclamide were 102 and 101% at 30 minutes, which gradually increased and after 180 min were found to be103 and 106% respectively. Interacting results shows that no remarkable drifts in the availabilities and no drift in retention time were observed (**Table 19**). However the results showed that no interaction occurred as there was no significant change in % availabilities of both drugs were observed by HPLC.

(mins)	CAP	MET	CAP	PGL	CAP	GLB
0	99.89	100.01	100.34	100.34	99.9	99
30	101	103	99.54	99.54	101.3	101
60	100.23	103.3	99.98	99.6	102.3	102.3
90	99.98	103.2	99.3	99.69	102.3	102.6
120	100.2	104	98.46	99.96	102	102
150	101.98	104.3	100.3	100.3	103.02	104.02
180	100.03	105.3	102	104	103	106.03

Table 19.
% availability of captopril and antidiabetic drugs by HPLC.

mins	LSP	MET	LSP	PGL	LSP	GLB
0	99.89	100.01	100.34	100.34	100	99.2
30	99.65	100.3	99.54	100.3	101.7	101.3
60	100.23	100.8	99.98	100.6	100.5	101.3
90	99.98	101.3	99.3	100.9	101.3	101.02
120	101.3	102.5	100.3	101.3	101.3	101
150	101.98	103.6	100.3	102.3	102.01	102.5
180	103.33	104.0	101.36	102.3	103	103.2

Table 20.
% Availability of lisinopril and antidiabetic drugs by HPLC.

3.4.3 Interaction of lisinopril with antidiabetic drugs by HPLC

In this study drugs were analyzed by measuring the area under curve (AUC), % recovery and considerable drift in retention time. Presence of metformin, pioglitazone and glibenclamide could also not assert any significant change in availability of lisinopril at 37°C. Availability of lisinopril with metformin was 103.33 at the end of experiment and that of metformin was 104.33%. In presence of pioglitazone and glibenclamide 100.3 and 102% of drug was available at the end of experiment and the availability of pioglitazone and glibenclamide were also not affected in presence of lisinopril. The obtained results showed that the NIDDMs and lisinopril do not affect *in-vitro* availability of each other at 37°C (**Table 20**).

4. Conclusions

The method described is simple, universal, convenient and reproducible simultaneous method that can be used to determine and quantify ACE inhibitors and antidiabetic drugs. Reliability, rapidness, simplicity, sensitivity, economical nature, good recovery and precision of this method give it an advantage over the other reported HPLC methods for the determination of ACE inhibitors and antidiabetic drugs. In summary, the proposed method can be used for drug analysis in routine quality control. In addition, this method has wide application in clinical research and pharmacokinetics drug interactions.

Conflict of interest

The authors declare no conflict of interest.

Author details

Safila Naveed* and Halima Sadia
Department of Pharmaceutical Chemistry, Faculty of Pharmacy, Jinnah University
for Women, Karachi, Pakistan

*Address all correspondence to: safila117@gmail.com

IntechOpen

References

[1] Bernstein KE, Martin BM, Edwards AS, Bernstein EA. Mouse angiotensin-converting enzyme is a protein composed of two homologous domains. Journal of Biological Chemistry. 1989 Jul 15;264(20):11945-51.

[2] Soubrier F, Alhenc-Gelas F, Hubert C, Allegrini J, John M, Tregear G, Corvol P. Two putative active centers in human angiotensin I-converting enzyme revealed by molecular cloning. Proceedings of the National Academy of Sciences. 1988 Dec 1;85(24):9386-90.

[3] Garcia-Sainz JA, Martinez-Alfaro M, Romero-Avila MT, Gonzalez-Espinosa C. Characterization of the AT1 angiotensin II receptor expressed in guinea pig liver. Journal of endocrinology. 1997 Jul 1;154(1):133-8.

[4] Ferreira SH. A bradykinin-potentiating factor (BPF) present in the venom of *Bothrops jararaca*. British journal of pharmacology and chemotherapy. 1965 Feb;24(1):163-9.

[5] Brar S, Ye F, James MT, Hemmelgarn B, Klarenbach S, Pannu N, Interdisciplinary Chronic Disease Collaboration. Association of angiotensin-converting enzyme inhibitor or angiotensin receptor blocker use with outcomes after acute kidney injury. JAMA internal medicine. 2018 Dec 1;178(12):1681-90.

[6] Dhull RS, Baracco R, Jain A, Mattoo TK. Pharmacologic treatment of pediatric hypertension. Current hypertension reports. 2016 Apr 1;18(4):32.

[7] Naveed S. Interaction Studies of ACE Inhibitors with Statins. Hyper-cholesterolemia. 2015 Sep 17:203.

[8] Rump LC, Baranova E, Okopien B, Weisskopf M, Kandra A, Ferber P. Coadministration of valsartan 160 and 320 mg and simvastatin 20 and 40 mg in patients with hypertension and hypercholesterolemia: a multicenter, 12-week, double-blind, double-dummy, parallel-group superiority study. Clinical therapeutics. 2008 Oct 1;30(10):1782-93.

[9] Sultana N, Arayne MS, Naveed S. Simultaneous determination of enalapril and statin's in pharmaceutical formulations by Rp-hplc. Journal of the Chilean Chemical Society. 2011;56(3): 734-7.

[10] Accary C, Hraoui-Bloquet S, Sadek R, Alameddine A, Fajloun Z, Desfontis JC, Mallem Y. The relaxant effect of the *Montivipera bornmuelleri* snake venom on vascular contractility. Journal of venom research. 2016;7:10.

[11] Ershov A, Petesburg S, Petesburg S, Petesburg S, Petesburg S. Synthesis of (2S, 4S)-2-Substituted-3-(3-Sulfanyl-propanoyl)-6-Oxohexahydro-pyrimidine-4-Carboxylic Acids as Potential Antihypertensive Drugs. Journal of Materials Science and Chemical Engineering. 2015;3(06):7.

[12] Sangshetti JN, Khan FA, Kulkarni AA, Arote R, Patil RH. Antileishmanial drug discovery: Comprehensive review of the last 10 years. Rsc Advances. 2015;5(41): 32376-415.

[13] Schoser B, Fong E, Geberhiwot T, Hughes D, Kissel JT, Madathil SC, Orlikowski D, Polkey MI, Roberts M, Tiddens HA, Young P. *Maximum* inspiratory pressure as a clinically meaningful trial endpoint for neuro-muscular diseases: a comprehensive review of the literature. Orphanet journal of rare diseases. 2017 Dec;12(1):1-2.

[14] Liliya L. Development of methodology for identification of captopril in medicines. Asian Journal of Pharmaceutics (AJP): Free full text

articles from Asian J Pharm. 2016 Sep 7;10(3).

[15] Bersanetti PA, Nogueira RF, Marcondes MF, Paiva PB, Juliano MA, Juliano L, Carmona AK, Zanotto FP. Characterization of angiotensin I-converting enzyme from anterior gills of the mangrove crab *Ucides cordatus*. International journal of biological macromolecules. 2015 Mar 1;74:304-9.

[16] Xiao F, Burns KD. Measurement of angiotensin converting enzyme 2 activity in biological fluid (ACE2). InHypertension 2017 (pp. 101-115). Humana Press, New York, NY.

[17] Abdulazeez MA, Kurfi BG. Isolation, partial purification and characterization of angiotensin converting enzyme from rat (*Rattus norvegicus*) lungs. Bayero Journal of Pure and Applied Sciences. 2016;9(2):24-9.

[18] Hong L, Lanying C. Purification and characterization of angiotensin converting enzyme. Zhongguo Sheng wu hua xue yu fen zi Sheng wu xue bao= Chinese Journal of Biochemistry and Molecular Biology. 2000 Jan 1;16(6): 788-92.

[19] Margalef M, Bravo FI, Arola-Arnal A, Muguerza B. Natural Angiotensin Converting Enzyme (ACE) Inhibitors with Antihypertensive Properties. Natural Products Targeting Clinically Relevant Enzymes. 2017 Oct 2:45-67.

[20] Drapak I, Kamenetska O, Perekhoda L, Sych I. Historical overview, development and new approaches in design of angiotensin converting enzyme inhibitors and angiotensin receptor antagonists. Part I. Scripta Scientifica Pharmaceutica. 2016 Apr 25;3(1):19-33.

[21] Ha GE, Chang OK, Jo SM, Han GS, Park BY, Ham JS, Jeong SG. Identification of antihypertensive peptides derived from low molecular weight casein hydrolysates generated during fermentation by *Bifidobacterium longum* KACC 91563. Korean journal for food science of animal resources. 2015;35(6):738.

[22] Borghi C, Ambrosioni E. A risk-benefit assessment of ACE inhibitor therapy post-myocardial infarction. Drug safety. 1996 May;14(5):277-87.

[23] Borghi C, Del Corso F, Faenza S, Cosentino E. ACE Inhibitor and Renin–Angiotensin System the Cornerstone of Therapy for Systolic Heart Failure. InACEi and ARBS in Hypertension and Heart Failure 2015 (pp. 41-72). Springer, Cham.

[24] Culley CM, DiBridge JN, Wilson Jr GL. Off-label use of agents for management of serious or life-threatening angiotensin converting enzyme inhibitor–induced angioedema. Annals of Pharmacotherapy. 2016 Jan;50(1):47-59.

[25] Singh Grewal A, Bhardwaj S, Pandita D, Lather V, Singh Sekhon B. Updates on aldose reductase inhibitors for management of diabetic complications and non-diabetic diseases. Mini Reviews in Medicinal Chemistry. 2016 Jan 1;16(2):120-62.

[26] Flaten HK, Monte AA. The pharmacogenomic and metabolomic predictors of ACE inhibitor and angiotensin II receptor blocker effectiveness and safety. Cardiovascular drugs and therapy. 2017 Aug;31(4):471-82.

[27] Mochel JP, Fink M, Peyrou M, Soubret A, Giraudel JM, Danhof M. Pharmacokinetic/pharmacodynamic modeling of renin-angiotensin aldosterone biomarkers following angiotensin-converting enzyme (ACE) inhibition therapy with benazepril in dogs. Pharmaceutical research. 2015 Jun;32(6):1931-46.

[28] Nithya R. An Investigation on the Incidence and Prevalence of Drug Related Outcomes in Hypertensive Patients on Ace Inhibitors (Doctoral dissertation, Swamy Vivekanandha College of Pharmacy, Tiruchengode).

[29] Boal AH, Smith DJ, McCallum L, Muir S, Touyz RM, Dominiczak AF, Padmanabhan S. Monotherapy with major antihypertensive drug classes and risk of hospital admissions for mood disorders. Hypertension. 2016 Nov;68(5):1132-8.

[30] Brewster LM, van Montfrans GA, Oehlers GP, Seedat YK. Systematic review: antihypertensive drug therapy in patients of African and South Asian ethnicity. Internal and emergency medicine. 2016 Apr 1;11(3):355-74.

[31] Oparil S, Schmieder RE. New approaches in the treatment of hypertension. Circulation research. 2015 Mar 13;116(6):1074-95.

[32] Lee RM, Dickhout JG, Sandow SL. Vascular structural and functional changes: their association with causality in hypertension: models, remodeling and relevance. Hypertension Research. 2017 Apr;40(4):311-23.

[33] Messerli FH, Rimoldi SF, Bangalore S. The transition from hypertension to heart failure: contemporary update. JACC: Heart Failure. 2017 Aug;5(8):543-51.

[34] Viazzi F, Bonino B, Cappadona F, Pontremoli R. Renin–angiotensin–aldosterone system blockade in chronic kidney disease: current strategies and a look ahead. Internal and emergency medicine. 2016 Aug;11(5):627-35.

[35] Diamond JA, Phillips RA. Hypertensive heart disease. Hypertension research. 2005 Mar;28(3):191-202.

[36] Joint National Committee on Detection, Treatment of High Blood Pressure, National High Blood Pressure Education Program. Coordinating Committee. Report of the joint national committee on detection, evaluation, and treatment of high blood pressure. National Heart, Lung, and Blood Institute, National High Blood Pressure Education Program.; 1995.

[37] Schmieder RE, Martus P, Klingbeil A. 781-6 Reversal of Left Ventricular Hypertrophy in Essential Hypertension: Meta-Analysis of Studies with High Scientific Quality. Journal of the American College of Cardiology. 1995 Feb 1;25(2):300A.

[38] Fogari R, Zoppi AN, Malamani GD, Marasi GI, Vanasia A, Villa G. Effects of different antihypertensive drugs on plasma fibrinogen in hypertensive patients. British journal of clinical pharmacology. 1995 May;39(5):471-6.

[39] Borghi C, Ambrosioni E. A risk-benefit assessment of ACE inhibitor therapy post-myocardial infarction. Drug safety. 1996 May;14(5):277-87.

[40] Murdoch DR, McMurray JJ. ACE inhibitors in acute myocardial infarction. Hospital medicine (London, England: 1998). 1998 Feb 1;59(2):111-5.

[41] Khan MS, Fonarow GC, Ahmed A, Greene SJ, Vaduganathan M, Khan H, Marti C, Gheorghiade M, Butler J. Dose of angiotensin-converting enzyme inhibitors and angiotensin receptor blockers and outcomes in heart failure: a meta-analysis. Circulation: Heart Failure. 2017 Aug;10(8):e003956.

[42] Supino P, Borer JS, Preibisz JJ, Herrold EM. VASODILATING DRUGS PROVIDE NO CLINICAL BENEFIT FOR PATIENTS WITH CHRONIC NONISCHEMIC MITRAL REGURGITATION. Journal of the American College of Cardiology. 2011 Apr 5;57(14S):E1384

[43] Hayek T. Effect of angiotensin converting enzyme inhibitors on LDL

lipid peroxidation and atherosclerosis progression in apo E deficient mice. Circulation. 1995;92:I-625.

[44] Ravid M, Lang R, Rachmani R, Lishner M. Long-term renoprotective effect of angiotensin-converting enzyme inhibition in non—insulin-dependent diabetes mellitus: a 7-year follow-up study. Archives of internal medicine. 1996 Feb 12;156(3):286-9.

[45] Chaturvedi N, Sjolie AK, Stephenson JM, Abrahamian H, Keipes M, Castellarin A, Rogulja-Pepeonik Z, Fuller JH, EUCLID Study Group. Effect of lisinopril on progression of retinopathy in normotensive people with type 1 diabetes. The Lancet. 1998 Jan 3;351(9095):28-31.

[46] Lewis EJ, Hunsicker LG, Bain RP, Rohde RD. The effect of angiotensin-converting-enzyme inhibition on diabetic nephropathy. New England Journal of Medicine. 1993 Nov 11;329(20):1456-62.

[47] Wang Z, do Carmo JM, Aberdein N, Zhou X, Williams JM, Da Silva AA, Hall JE. Synergistic interaction of hypertension and diabetes in promoting kidney injury and the role of endoplasmic reticulum stress. Hypertension. 2017 May;69(5):879-91.

[48] Calò LA, Davis PA, Rigato M, Sgarabotto L. Angiotensin-converting enzyme inhibitors, angiotensin II type 1 receptor blockers and risk of COVID 19: information from Bartter's and Gitelman's syndromes patients. Journal of hypertension. 2020 Jul 1;38(7):1386.

[49] Messerli FH, Bangalore S, Bavishi C, Rimoldi SF. Angiotensin-converting enzyme inhibitors in hypertension: to use or not to use?. Journal of the American College of Cardiology. 2018 Apr 3;71(13):1474-82.

[50] Alderman CP. Adverse effects of the angiotensin-converting enzyme inhibitors. Annals of Pharmacotherapy. 1996 Jan;30(1):55-61.

[51] Khalil ME, Basher AW, Brown EJ, Alhaddad IA. A remarkable medical story: benefits of angiotensin-converting enzyme inhibitors in cardiac patients. Journal of the American College of Cardiology. 2001 Jun 1;37(7):1757-64.

[52] Johnston CI. Angiotensin converting enzyme inhibitors in the treatment of hypertension. InIUPHAR 9th International Congress of Pharmacology 1984 (pp. 105-110). Palgrave, London.

[53] Gilman AG. Goodman and Gilman's the pharmacological basis of therapeutics.

[54] Ravid D, Lishner M, Lang R, Ravid M. Angiotensin-converting enzyme inhibitors and cough: a prospective evaluation in hypertension and in congestive heart failure. The Journal of Clinical Pharmacology. 1994 Nov;34(11):1116-20.

[55] Zalawadiya SK, Sethi S, Loe S, Kumar S, Tchokonte R, Shi D, Adam AK, May EJ. Unique case of presumed lisinopril-induced hepatotoxicity. American Journal of Health-System Pharmacy. 2010 Aug 15;67(16):1354-6.

[56] Harrison B, Laidlaw S, Reilly J. Fatal aplastic anaemia associated with lisinopril. The Lancet. 1995 Jul 22; 346(8969):247-8.

[57] Dzau VJ. Renal effects of angiotensin-converting enzyme inhibition in cardiac failure. American journal of kidney diseases: the official journal of the National Kidney Foundation. 1987 Jul 1;10(1 Suppl 1):74-80.

[58] Murphy BF, Whitworth JA, Kincaid-Smith P. Renal insufficiency with combinations of angiotensin converting enzyme inhibitors and diuretics. British medical journal (Clinical research ed.). 1984 Mar 17;288(6420):844.

[59] Navis G, Faber HJ, de Zeeuw D, de Jong PE. ACE inhibitors and the kidney. Drug safety. 1996 Sep;15(3):200-11.

[60] Messerli FH, Bangalore S, Julius S. Risk/benefit assessment of β-blockers and diuretics precludes their use for first-line therapy in hypertension. Circulation. 2008 May 20;117(20): 2706-15.

[61] McMurray J, Matthews DM. Consequences of fluid loss in patients treated with ACE inhibitors. Postgraduate medical journal. 1987 May 1;63 (739):385-7.

[62] Israili ZH, Hall WD. Cough and angioneurotic edema associated with angiotensin-converting enzyme inhibitor therapy: a review of the literature and pathophysiology. Annals of internal medicine. 1992 Aug 1;117(3):234-42.

[63] Lindgren BR, Andersson RG. Angiotensin-converting enzyme inhibitors and their influence on inflammation, bronchial reactivity and cough. Medical toxicology and adverse drug experience. 1989 Oct;4(5):369-80.

[64] Sabroe RA, Black AK. Angiotensin–converting enzyme (ACE) inhibitors and angio–oedema. British Journal of Dermatology. 1997 Feb;136(2):153-8.

[65] Chin HL, Buchan DA. Severe angioedema after long-term use of an angiotensin-converting enzyme inhibitor. Annals of internal medicine. 1990 Feb 15;112(4):312-3.

[66] Hameed MS, Patel AV, Bertino JS. Delayed angiotensin-converting enzyme inhibitor-induced angioedema. Hospital Physician. 2006 Feb;42(2):33.

[67] Boodoo S, De Gannes K, Maharaj S, Pandey S, Ahmad A, Dhingra S. Angiotensin-Converting Enzyme (ACE) Induced Angioedema: A Case Report. International Journal of Toxicological

and Pharmacological Research. 2014; 6(4):121-2.

[68] Wood SM, Mann RD, Rawlins MD. Angio-oedema and urticaria associated with angiotensin converting enzyme inhibitors. British medical journal (Clinical research ed.). 1987 Jan 10;294(6564):91.

[69] Sedman AB, Kershaw DB, Bunchman TE. Invited Review Recognition and management of angiotensin converting enzyme inhibitor fetopathy. Pediatric Nephrology. 1995 Jun;9(3):382-5.

[70] Pryde PG, Sedman AB, Nugent CE, Barr M. Angiotensin-converting enzyme inhibitor fetopathy. Journal of the American Society of Nephrology. 1993 Mar 1;3(9):1575-82.

[71] Boras VV, Brailo V, Juras DV. Ramipril Induced Burning Mouth Symptoms. Annual Research & Review in Biology. 2014 Jul 17:3945-8.

[72] Obergassel L, Carlsson J, Tebbe U. ACE inhibitor-associated interstitial lung infiltrates. Deutsche medizinische Wochenschrift (1946). 1995 Sep 1; 120(38):1273-7.

[73] Verresen L, Waer M, Vanrenterghem Y, Michielsen P. Angiotensin-converting-enzyme inhibitors and anaphylactoid reactions to high-flux membrane dialysis. The Lancet. 1990 Dec 1;336(8727):1360-2.

[74] Verresen L, Waer M, Vanrenterghem Y, Michielsen P. Angiotensin-converting-enzyme inhibitors and anaphylactoid reactions to high-flux membrane dialysis. The Lancet. 1990 Dec 1;336(8727):1360-2.

[75] Shotan A, Widerhorn J, Hurst A, Elkayam U. Risks of angiotensin-converting enzyme inhibition during pregnancy: experimental and clinical evidence, potential mechanisms, and

recommendations for use. The American journal of medicine. 1994 May 1;96(5):451-6.

[76] Grégoire JP, Moisan J, Guibert R, Ciampi A, Milot A, Côté I, Gaudet M. Tolerability of antihypertensive drugs in a community-based setting. Clinical therapeutics. 2001 May 1;23(5):715-26.

[77] Salmon P, Brown M. Renal artery stenosis and peripheral vascular disease: implications for ACE inhibitor therapy. The Lancet. 1990 Aug 4;336(8710):321.

[78] Pfaadt M. The Physician Desk Reference (PDR) Family Guide. Home Healthcare Now. 1996 Oct 1;14(10):832-3.

[79] Augenstein WL, Kulig KW, Rumack BH. Captopril overdose resulting in hypotension. JAMA. 1988 Jun 10;259(22):3302-5.

[80] Kulig K, Augenstein WL, Rumack BH. Captopril Overdose and Hypotension-Reply. JAMA. 1988 Nov 4;260(17):2508

[81] Waeber B, Nussberger J, Brunner HR. Self poisoning with enalapril. British medical journal (Clinical research ed.). 1984 Jan 28;288(6413):287.

[82] Belay TW. Lisinopril overdose. Reactions. 2014 Mar;1491:23-8.

[83] Trilli LE, Johnson KA. Lisinopril overdose and management with intravenous angiotensin II. Annals of Pharmacotherapy. 1994 Oct;28(10):1165-8.

[84] Newby DE, Lee MR, Gray AJ, Boon NA. Enalapril overdose and the corrective effect of intravenous angiotensin II. British journal of clinical pharmacology. 1995 Jul;40(1):103.

[85] Enalapril overdose treated with angiotensin infusion, Lancet

[86] Koopmans PP, Van Megen T, Thien T, Gribnau FW. The interaction between indomethacin and captopril or enalapril in healthy volunteers. Journal of internal medicine. 1989 Sep;226(3):139-42.

[87] Bainbridge AD, MacFadyen RJ, Lees KR, Reid JL. A study of the acute pharmacodynamic interaction of ramipril and felodipine in normotensive subjects. British journal of clinical pharmacology. 1991 Feb;31(2):148-53.

[88] Horvath AM, Blake DS, Ferry JJ, Sedman AJ, Colburn WA. PROPRANOLOL DOES NOT INFLUENCE QUINAPRIL PHARMACOKINETICS IN HEALTHY-VOLUNTEERS. InJournal of Clinical Pharmacology 1987 Sep 1 (Vol. 27, No. 9, pp. 719-719). 227 EAST WASHINGTON SQ, PHILADELPHIA, PA 19106: LIPPINCOTT-RAVEN PUBL.

[89] Casato M, Pucillo LP, Leoni M, di Lullo L, Gabrielli A, Sansonno D, Dammacco F, Danieli G, Bonomo L. Granulocytopenia after combined therapy with interferon and angiotensin-converting enzyme inhibitors: evidence for a synergistic hematologic toxicity. The American journal of medicine. 1995 Oct 1;99(4):386-91.

[90] Healey LA, Backes MB. Nitritoid reactions and angiotensin-converting-enzyme inhibitors. The New England journal of medicine. 1989 Sep 1; 321(11):763

[91] Dercksen MW, Hoekman K, Visser JJ, ten Bokkel Huinink WW, Pinedo HM, Wagstaff J. Hypotension induced by interleukin-3 in patients on angiotensin-converting enzyme inhibitors. Lancet. 1995;345:448.

[92] D'costa DF, Basu SK, Gunasekera NP. ACE inhibitors and diuretics causing hypokalaemia. The British journal of clinical practice. 1990 Jan 1;44(1):26-7.

[93] Toussaint CA, Masselink A, Gentges A, Wambach G, Bönner G.

Interference of different ACE-inhibitors with the diuretic action of furosemide and hydrochlorothiazide. Klinische Wochenschrift. 1989 Nov 1;67(22):1138-46.

[94] Shionoiri H. Pharmacokinetic drug interactions with ACE inhibitors. Clinical pharmacokinetics. 1993 Jul;25(1):20-58.

[95] Amir O, Hassan Y, Sarriff A, Awaisu A, Aziz NA, Ismail O. Incidence of risk factors for developing hyperkalemia when using ACE inhibitors in cardiovascular diseases. Pharmacy world & science. 2009 Jun;31(3):387-93.

[96] Good CB, McDermott L, McCloskey B. Diet and serum potassium in patients on ACE inhibitors. JAMA. 1995 Aug 16;274(7):538

[97] Golik A, Zaidenstein R, Dishi V, Blatt A, Cohen N, Cotter G, Berman S, Weissgarten J. Effects of captopril and enalapril on zinc metabolism in hypertensive patients. Journal of the American College of Nutrition. 1998 Feb 1;17(1):75-8.

[98] Baba T, Tomiyama T, Takebe K. Enhancement by an ACE Inhibitor of First-Dose Hypotension Caused by an Alpha1-Blocker. The New England journal of medicine. 1990 Apr 26;322(17).

[99] Lee SC, Park SW, Kim DK, Lee SH, Hong KP. Iron supplementation inhibits cough associated with ACE inhibitors. Hypertension. 2001 Aug 1;38(2):166-70.

[100] Campbell NR, Hasinoff BB. Iron supplements: a common cause of drug interactions. British journal of clinical pharmacology. 1991 Mar;31(3):251-5.

[101] Herings RM, De Boer A, Leufkens HG, Porsius A, Stricker BC. Hypoglycaemia associated with use of inhibitors of angiotensin converting enzyme. The Lancet. 1995 May 13;345(8959):1195-8.

[102] Morris AD, Boyle DI, McMahon AD, Pearce H, Evans JM, Newton RW, Jung RT, MacDonald TM, Darts/Memo Collaboration. ACE inhibitor use is associated with hospitalization for severe hypoglycemia in patients with diabetes. Diabetes Care. 1997 Sep 1;20(9):1363-7.

[103] Gossmann J, Kachel HG, Schoeppe WI, Scheuermann EH. Anemia in renal transplant recipients caused by concomitant therapy with azathioprine and angiotensin-converting enzyme inhibitors. Transplantation. 1993 Sep 1;56(3):585-9.

[104] Jensen K, Bunemann L, Riisager S, Thomsen LJ. Cerebral blood flow during anaesthesia: influence of pretreatment with metoprolol or captopril. BJA: British Journal of Anaesthesia. 1989 Mar 1;62(3):321-3.

[105] Kalra S, Gupta Y. Sulfonylureas. JPMA. The Journal of the Pakistan Medical Association. 2015 Jan 1;65(1):101-4.

[106] Malaisse WJ. Gliquidone contributes to improvement of type 2 diabetes mellitus management. Drugs in R & D. 2006 Nov;7(6):331-7.

[107] O'Byrne S, Feely J. Effects of drugs on glucose tolerance in non-insulin-dependent diabetics (Part II). Drugs. 1990 Aug;40(2):203-19.

[108] Porta V, Schramm SG, Kano EK, Koono EE, Armando YP, Fukuda K, dos Reis Serra CH. HPLC-UV determination of metformin in human plasma for application in pharmacokinetics and bioequivalence studies. Journal of Pharmaceutical and biomedical analysis. 2008 Jan 7;46(1):143-7.

[109] Arayne MS, Sultana N, Zuberi MH. Development and validation of RP-HPLC method for the analysis of metformin. Pak J Pharm Sci. 2006 Jul 1;19(3):231-5.

[110] Wang Y, Tang Y, Gu J, Fawcett JP, Bai X. Rapid and sensitive liquid chromatography–tandem mass spectrometric method for the quantitation of metformin in human plasma. Journal of Chromatography B. 2004 Sep 5;808(2): 215-9.

[111] Amini H, Ahmadiani A, Gazerani P. Determination of metformin in human plasma by high-performance liquid chromatography. Journal of Chromatography B. 2005 Sep 25;824(1-2):319-22.

[112] AbuRuz S, Millership J, McElnay J. The development and validation of liquid chromatography method for the simultaneous determination of metformin and glipizide, gliclazide, glibenclamide or glimperide in plasma. Journal of Chromatography B. 2005 Mar 25;817(2):277-86.

[113] Vasudevan M, Ravi J, Ravisankar S, Suresh B. Ion-pair liquid chromatography technique for the estimation of metformin in its multicomponent dosage forms. Journal of pharmaceutical and biomedical analysis. 2001 Apr 1;25(1):77-84.

[114] Shaheen O, Othman S, Jalal I, Awidi A, Al-Turk W. Comparison of pharmacokinetics and pharmaco-dynamics of a conventional and a new rapidly dissolving glibenclamide preparation. International journal of pharmaceutics. 1987 Aug 1;38(1-3): 123-31.

[115] Kaminski L, Degenhardt M, Ermer J, Feußner C, Höwer-Fritzen H, Link P, Renger B, Tegtmeier M, Wätzig H. Efficient and economic HPLC performance qualification. Journal of pharmaceutical and biomedical analysis. 2010 Feb 5;51(3):557-64.

[116] Yao J, Shi YQ, Li ZR, Jin SH. Development of a RP-HPLC method for screening potentially counterfeit anti-diabetic drugs. Journal of Chromatography B. 2007 Jun 15;853(1-2):254-9.

[117] Sharma N, Mishra A, Kumar R, Sharma S, Bhandari A. Second Derivative Spectrophotometric method for the estimation of Metformin Hydrochloride in Bulk and in Tablet Doage Form. Int J Pharma & Pharmace Sci. 2011;3(4):333-5.

[118] Holman RR, Turner RC, Pickup J, Williams G. Textbook of diabetes. by Pickup J., Williams G., Blackwell, Oxford. 1991:467-9.

[119] Erdmann E. Microalbuminuria as a marker of cardiovascular risk in patients with type 2 diabetes. International journal of cardiology. 2006 Feb 15;107(2):147-53.

[120] Triplitt C. Drug interactions of medications commonly used in diabetes. Diabetes Spectrum. 2006 Oct 1;19(4):202-11.

[121] Cheung BM. Blockade of the renin-angiotensin system. Hong Kong Medical Journal. 2002.

[122] Reduce CB. Diabetes Risk In Hispanic Patients. ScienceDaily (May 22, 2006).

[123] Leichter SB, Thomas S. Combination medications in diabetes care: an opportunity that merits more attention. Clinical Diabetes. 2003 Oct 1;21(4):175-8.

[124] Ibsen H, Olsen MH, Wachtell K, Borch-Johnsen K, Lindholm LH, Mogensen CE, Dahlöf B, Devereux RB, de Faire U, Fyhrquist F, Julius S. Reduction in albuminuria translates to reduction in cardiovascular events in hypertensive patients: losartan intervention for endpoint reduction in hypertension study. Hypertension. 2005 Feb 1;45(2):198-202.

[125] Scheen AJ. Drug interactions of clinical importance with

antihyperglycaemic agents. Drug safety.
2005 Jul;28(7):601-31.

[126] Mitra SK, Sundaram R,
Venkataranganna MV, Gopumadhavan S.
Pharmacokinetic interaction of
Diabecon (D-400) with rifampicin and
nifedipine. European journal of drug
metabolism and pharmacokinetics. 1999
Mar 1;24(1):79-82.

Chapter 6

Combined Effect of Metformin and Statin

Sabu Mandumpal Chacko and Priya Thambi Thekkekara

Abstract

Diabetes mellitus (DM) is considered a risk factor for the development of coronary artery disease (CAD). Metformin, an anti-diabetic drug, has been shown to lower the cardiovascular events in pre-clinical and clinical studies. Many research articles suggests that metformin has a protective effect on CAD beyond its hypoglycemic effects. Patients with diabetes type 2 have an increased risk for cardiovascular disease and commonly use combination therapy consisting of the anti-diabetic drug metformin and a cholesterol-lowering statin. Statins have been found to be a safe and effective approach to reduce serum low density lipoprotein cholesterol (LDL-C) levels, which is the cornerstone for primary and secondary prevention of atherosclerosis. However, regular statin monotherapy in some patients may not be sufficient to achieve a therapeutic LDL-C. It has been reported that statins increased the incidence of new-onset diabetes in a dose dependent manner especially in women, the elderly, or in the presence of a family history of type 2 diabetes (T2D) and Asian ethnicity. The molecular mechanisms contributed to antioxidation, anti-inflammation, and anti-apoptosis. In this chapter, we aimed to investigate whether the combined administration of metformin and atorvastatin could achieve superior protective effects on different disease treatment purpose and to elucidate its molecular mechanisms of the combinations.

Keywords: combination therapy, metformin, statins, diabetes mellitus, clinical studies

1. Introduction

World Health Organization (WHO) defines diabetes mellitus as a metabolic disorder of multiple etiologies characterized by chronic hyperglycemia with alterations of carbohydrate absorption, fat and protein metabolism. DM is one of the four major non-communicable diseases along with cardiovascular disease (CVD), cancer and chronic respiratory diseases. Once a disease of affluence, it is now increasingly common among the poor countries [1]. The morbidity and mortality associated with DM arises from minor and macrovascular complications, ischemic heart disease (IHD) and peripheral vascular disease (PVD) [2]. Metformin acts by several mechanisms of action but the major mechanism is inhibiting hepatic gluconeogenesis [3]. The drug may antagonize the action of glucagon, and reduces fasting blood glucose (FBG) [4]. In addition, metformin increases insulin action at target sites, increases peripheral glucose uptake, enhances fatty acid oxidation and reduces glucose absorption from gastrointestinal tract [5]. Diabetes mellitus and statins have a complex association and are the attention of patient and healthcare debate. Statins are widely used as a part of diabetes mellitus care due to that patients with DM have a greater CVD [6]. At the early stage, the heart only showed transcriptional and metabolic altercations, including enhanced inflammation, oxidative stress, depletion of antioxidant proteins, and changes in energy metabolism. Use of statins in diabetes is a controversial when compared with metformin. Although the potential detrimental effects of statin on muscle and liver have been known for a long time, new concerns have emerged regarding the risk of new onset diabetes (NOM). This often leads to discontinuation of statin, non-adherence to therapy, or concerns correlating with initiating statin therapy.

There are several CVD risk factors, including hypertension, dyslipidemia, diabetes mellitus (DM), smoking and obesity, as well as platelet dysfunction. Certain drugs are currently available for treating these risk factors, whereas drug combinations are frequently needed to achieve therapeutic goals especially in hypertension, DM and coronary heart disease (CHD). Based on these considerations our objectives were 1) to assess whether combination therapy shows clinical effectiveness for cognition and functional benefits in a well-characterized prospective cohort of patients with T2DM treated over years with metformin; 2) to determine the magnitude and duration of benefit; 3) to characterize the long-term treatment of patients who receive combination therapy compared to those who were never treated with statins and those who only received metformin as monotherapy; and 4) to use modeling methods to make predictions about the mechanism and clinical course in different treatment groups and dose levels.

Both metformin and statins thus act on glucose—as well as lipid metabolism which is why metformin–statin combination therapy is prescribed to many T2DM patients. Since both drugs act on glucose as well as lipid metabolism, it is important to understand in detail the interactions between metformin and statin mechanism of action on treatment design with different dose level and optimal safety/efficacy profiles. This chapter is therefore designed to provide insight in the mechanism of combined effect of statin/metformin not only on DM and CVD but also with different types of cancer and other diseases. This chapter also explain the interaction of both drugs on preclinical and clinical studies to determine an optimal dosing strategy of both drugs.

2. Metformin

Metformin is an oral antidiabetic drug, discovered in 1922, came on the market as late as 1979 [7]. The drug is belongs to the biguanide classification and derivative from guanidine found in *Galega officinalis*. It is available in different formulations based on its duration of action like immediate-release, extended release and delayed-release metformin [8, 9]. The latter two forms were developed to expand the absorption of metformin along the gut. Metformin administration in 30 min before a meal produced highest therapeutic efficacy in lowering postprandial hyperglycemia [10].

2.1 Metformin absorption and distribution

Oral administration of metformin transported into the small intestine across the apical membrane into the enterocytes via several transporter proteins. The main proteins are the plasma monoamine transporter (PMAT; SLC29A4), organic cation transporter 1 (OCT1; SLC22A1) and serotonin transporter protein (SERT; SLC6A4) [11].

Metformin accumulated majorly in the intestine, and in the stomach, liver, kidney and lesser extent in muscle. The accumulation of metformin in intestine and stomach is because of these organs are most exposed to high concentrations of metformin after oral administration. A recent study confirmed the high metformin levels are accumulated in these organs [12]. These concentrations are tenfold higher than metformin concentrations in the liver, indicating that the intestine is probably an important site of action. In fact, the metformin effects in the intestine may be rather different than the effects in the liver. The concentration of metformin in human jejunum has been shown to be 30 to 300 fold greater than in plasma, and earlier studies demonstrating accumulation of metformin in the intestinal mucosa. Metformin navigates to the liver via the portal vein and is taken up predominantly by organic cation transporter (OCT1) as well as by Thiamine transporter (THTR-2). In this chapter, the effects of metformin on the lipid metabolism are highlighted, thereby creating a special focus on the effects on lipids related to the activation of AMPK by metformin (**Figure 1**) [13].

Metformin is transported into hepatocytes mainly via OCT1, and inhibited the mitochondrial respiratory chain (complex I) through a currently unknown mechanism(s). The deficit in energy production is balanced by reducing gluconeogenesis in the liver. This is mediated in two main ways. First, a decrease in ATP and a concomitantly increase in AMP concentration. Second, increased AMP levels function as a key signaling mediator to (1) allosterically inhibit cAMP–PKA signaling by suppression of adenylatecyclase, (2) allosterically inhibit FBPase, (3) activates AMPK. This leads to inhibition of gluconeogenesis (1 and 2) and lipid/cholesterol synthesis (3).

Metformin is present for over 99% in the mono protonated form in all tissues of the body except in the stomach. The sparse data showed, that metformin is mostly distributed in the cytosolic fraction (~ 70%) of rat hepatic cells compared to mixed membranes (12%), nucleus (~ 5%), and mitochondrial and lysosomal fractions (8%). A low binding affinity of metformin to mitochondrial membranes was seen, and this may be because of the two methyl groups present in metformin structure [14]. Previous study concludes that, the mitochondrial membrane

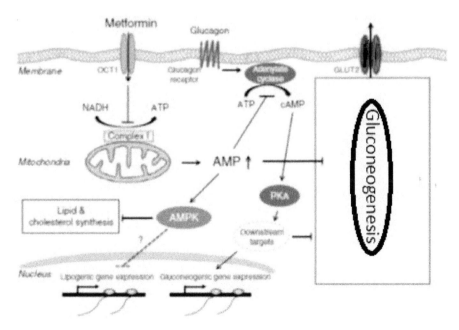

Figure 1.
Schematic diagram of the anti-hyperglycaemic action of metformin on the liver cell.

potential may promote entry of metformin (positively charged) [15], which will then concentrate inside the mitochondria (negatively charged) [16]. Molecular modeling of the metformin distribution and validation study confirmed the presence of high concentrations of the drug in the endoplasmic reticulum (ER) and in the mitochondria, based on its membrane potential [17].

2.2 Metformin mechanisms on glucose and lipid metabolism

The main mechanisms of metformin involved in decreasing the endogenous glucose production and plasma glucose have all been extensively reviewed and critically discussed in earlier studies [18]. Metformin shows beneficial effects on the glucose and lipid metabolism, even though the pathways are not fully understood [19]. In patient studies, the variations of metformin efficacy may be due to the presence of responders and non-responders to the drug treatment [20], racial and ethnic background [21], and personal variation in the adaptation of metformin treatment. Sonne et al., [22] proposed a pathway inducing reduction of LDL cholesterol by the. Inhibition of the intestinal absorption of bile acids is caused by metformin. It causes an increased synthesis of bile acids in the liver, and cholesterol is used for this process [23], thereby causing a decreased amount of cholesterol in the hepatic cells. Upregulation of the LDL-C receptor may increase the uptake of lipoproteins, to restore a sufficient level of cholesterol in the liver. Hence, metformin indirectly decrease the LDL-C concentration and plasma total cholesterol concentrations.

2.3 (In)-direct effects of metformin on β cells

A decreased β cell mass is an important factor in the development of T2DM. High glucose and FFA induce damaging effects on β cells (e.g. decreased insulin secretion and β cell mass) [24]. It is therefore of interest to consider possible beneficial effects of metformin on β cell function. Lipase and amylase are secreted by the pancreas and are often measured to monitor the condition of the pancreas. There were no changes observed in the enzyme levels, and the pancreas volume when metformin (1950 mg/day) was given to T2DM patients for 24 weeks. This works suggesting that metformin does not repair damaged β cells [25].

3. Statin

Statins, block an enzyme called HMG-CoA reductase (3-hydroxy-3-methylglutaryl coenzyme A reductase) that is involved in the synthesis of mevalonate, a naturally occurring substance that is then used by the body to make cholesterol. By inhibiting this enzyme, LDL-cholesterol and cholesterol production is decreased. Statins also increase the number of LDL receptors on liver cells, which increases the uptake and breakdown of LDL-cholesterol. Most of the effects of statins, including the blocking of the HMG-CoA reductase enzyme occur in the liver. Many research have shown that elevated levels of total cholesterol, LDL-cholesterol, triglycerides, and apolipoprotein B increase a person's risk of developing heart disease or having a stroke.

3.1 Classification of statins and its general source

Statins are classified based on different criteria, including: 1) how they are obtained, 2) liver metabolism, 3) physicochemical properties, and 4) specific activity. Some of the statins are obtained after fungal fermentation: lovastatin, pravastatin and simvastatin, others by synthesis: fluvastatin, atorvastatin, and cerivastatin. Only five statins are, at this moment, in clinical use: lovastatin, simvastatin, pravastatin, atorvastatin and fluvastatin. Pravastatin is extremely hydrophilic, fluvastatin has intermediate characteristics, lovastatin, simvastatin, atorvastatin and cerivastatin are hydrophobic.

3.2 General uses of statins

- Statins differ in their potency at lowering total cholesterol, triglycerides, LDL-cholesterol, or increasing HDL-cholesterol; their propensity for drug interactions; and their reported safety in people with kidney disease.

- Reduce a person's risk of having a heart attack or stroke or developing angina

- Reduce the risk of further heart disease in people with type 2 diabetes or coronary artery disease.

- Simvastatin and atorvastatin produce the greatest percentage change in LDL cholesterol levels. Fluvastatin and atorvastatin are also preferred in hypocholesteremic patients with kidney disease.

- Pravastatin and fluvastatin have a lower risk of drug interactions because they are not metabolized by cytochrome p450 3A4.

- Pitavastatin has a similar effectiveness to atorvastatin but reportedly produces greater increases in HDL-cholesterol that are sustained over the long-term. It is effective at low dosages and has minimal drug interactions.

3.3 Statins mechanism on glucose and lipid lowering metabolism

Statins are a major class of drugs that decrease plasma cholesterol levels and are prescribed as first choice to patients suffering from CVD [26]. Simvastatin and atorvastatin are often given as a first choice to patients with cardiovascular risk factors/cardiovascular disease. In earlier studies reported that low dose (20 mg/day) of atorvastatin given to patients with myocardial infarction showed improved lipid, adipokine, and pro-inflammatory markers and decreased insulin resistance. Higher dose (40 mg/day) of atorvastatin showed hyperglycemia, increased leptin levels and ghrelin deficiency [27, 28] in diabetic patient. It was also discovered that the reduction in LDL-C by statins is an important indicator of increased T2DM risk [29]. Genetic factors and/orange-related factors could as well lead to the development of T2DM during statin treatment.

Several mechanisms possibly involved in the effect of statins on glucose metabolism are summarized in **Figure 2**. Statin signaling pathway that stimulates endogenous glucose production (EGP) by activation of gluconeogenic genes in human liver cells. Statin activates the pregnaneX receptor (PXR) in the cytoplasm. Many functions are exerts by PXR, such as the stimulation of the expression of proteins involved in regulation of hepatic glucose and removal of xenobiotics, and lipid metabolism [17].

3.4 Effects of statins in the β cell of pancreas

Statin mechanism may contribute to a decreased insulin secretion in the β cell, possibly contributing to the progress of T2DM. The upregulation of LDL-C receptor seen upon inhibition of HMG-CoA reductase are one of the directly

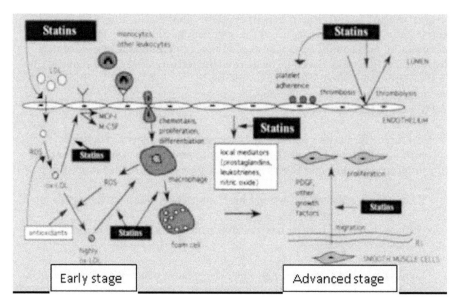

Figure 2.
Hypercholesterolemia enhance the entry of LDL particles into sub endothelial space at lesion-prone arterial sites. Monocyte chemotactic protein-1 (MCP-1) and oxidized-LDL act as chemoattractants to direct accumulation of monocytes and their migration to the subendothelial space, where monocytes undergo phenotypic transformation into macrophages. Oxygen free radicals concurrently modify LDL. Oxidatively modified LDL is taken up by nondownregulating macrophage receptors to form lipid-rich foam cells. The foam cells develop into fatty streaks that is the, precursor of atherosclerotic plaques. Statins exhibit pleiotropic effects on many components of atherosclerosis that accompany hypercholesterolemia, abnormal endothelial function and including platelet coagulation abnormalities, and determinants of plaque thrombogenicity such as plaque inflammation and proliferation.

affected processes, which results in increased uptake of plasma LDL-C into the β cell [30]. The increased amount of cholesterol within the cell causes interference with translocation of glucokinase, to the mitochondria [31]. A decreased glucose transporter (GLUT2) expression level was observed in simvastatin treated mouse MIN6 cells which resulted in a reduction of ATP levels. This may be the mechanism of inhibition of the KATP channel closure, membrane depolarization and calcium channel opening all leading to reduced insulin secretion [32]. Inhibition of the ATP-dependent potassium channel, depolarization and the decreased influx of intracellular calcium, and calcium concentrations were observed and were related to a decreased insulin secretion. In an ex vivo study, intracellular calcium levels were not affected even though intact with single-islets were treated with simvastatin [33]. Statin treatment may cause inactivation of Ras and Rho molecules, hence the activation and membrane translocalization of GLUT-4 is inhibited. Experiments with atorvastatin treatment in mouse adipocytes confirmed that GLUT-4 located on the plasma membrane moved to the cytosol during treatment and this may result in an increased insulin resistance [34].

3.5 Statins on cancer

Since 1959, evidence from many studies had revealed that there was an association between T2DM and cancer, and patients who had T2DM were more likely to be diagnosed with cancer than patients who had not [35, 36]. A lot of evidence has also shown its beneficial effects in cancers, including prostate, breast, lung, and colorectal cancers [37]. Experimental results in vitro have suggested the effect of statins on growth, migration, apoptosis, and autophagy of cancer cells [38, 39]. The data from in vivo cell culture studies, statins may act as a preventive drug for hepatocellular carcinoma, malignant glioma and bladder cancer [40]. However, the role of statins on the incidence of cancer in patients with T2DM has not been well documented. Fei et al., [41] performed a meta-analysis to evaluate the impact of different types of statins on the risk of cancers with T2DM.The study was systematically searched with the Cochrane Library, PubMed, Embase, and Wanfang databases from January 1999 to March 2017. A pairwise meta-analysis used to estimate the pooled ratios (ORs) and 95% confidence intervals (CIs). NMA was performed to compare different types of statins. In pairwise meta-analysis result showed that, the incidence of cancer in T2DM patients was reduced when simvastatin, atorvastatin, pravastatin, fluvastatin, lovastatin, rosuvastatin, and pitavastatin were used. The analyses suggest that rosuvastatin may be more effective than others.

4. Combination therapy of metformin and atorvastatin

4.1 On antidiabetic activity-preclinical studies

Previous studies on diabetic rats (200–220 g) reported that after 2 weeks of metformin–atorvastatin combination therapy (500 mg metformin and 20 mg atorvastatin per 70 kg body weight), reduced blood glucose, lipid-lowering effects, and reduced in elevated oxidative stress, and positive effects on cardiovascular hypertrophy occurred [42]. The reduction of oxidative stress and liver protection (blood analysis and liver histology studies, e.g. CRP, TNF-α, IL-6, protein carbonyl levels) was also seen in T2DM rats treated with metformin and atorvastatin [43].

Statins consistently showed a protective role in the setting of diabetes cardio-myopathy (DCM) due to their roles of anti-inflammation, anti-oxidation, and antiapoptosis effects [44]. In previous animal experiments, statins could prevent DCM by all evicting left ventricular dysfunction and inhibiting myocardial fibrosis through anti-apoptosis and anti-inflammation pathways. It seems that statins may facilitate the onset of diabetes by impacting peripheral insulin sensitivity and islet b-cell function, while statins can effectively modify the promotive factors and promoting DCM, including inflammation and oxidative stress, thereby protecting the heart against diabetic conditions [45].

4.2 On Antiatherosclerogenic activity-preclinical studies

An animal study was designed to evaluate the effectiveness safety and mecha-nism of an atorvastatin/metformin combination therapy in a rabbit atherosclerosis model induced by a high-cholesterol diet. At the end of the experiment, all rabbits were sacrificed by injection of an overdose of sodium pentobarbital solution and the aortas were separated from the surrounding tissues. From the initiation of the aortic arch, 0.5 cm sections were excised for paraffin treatment [46] and the remain-ing aortas were soaked in 4%paraformaldehyde and then stained with Oil Red O solution, to evaluate the atherosclerotic lesion area of the aorta by image-processing software (ImageJ). One portion stained with hematoxylin and eosin (H&E) before quantification using ImageJ software. In an animal study 12-week high-cholesterol diet induced a significant increase in atherosclerotic lesion area in rabbits in the control (Ctrl) group; after 10 weeks of atorvastatin or metformin treatment, the atherosclerotic lesion area was significantly reduced by 51% and 35%, respectively.

Atorvastatin/metformin combination therapy resulted in an 80% reduction of atherosclerotic plaques compared with the control group. The combination therapy showed which was more effectively than each monotherapy. Compared with control group, the treatment of atorvastatin or metformin significantly reduced the lesion size by 68% and 42%, respectively, while atorvastatin/metformin combination therapy further reduced atherosclerotic lesion size by 86%. It was reported that large HDL is inversely associated with cardiovascular disease [47]. The results suggest that atorvastatin and metformin combination therapy is superior to atorvastatin monotherapy for the treatment of athero-sclerosis and the underlying mechanisms might be associated with cholesterol efflux in macrophages. The study results demonstrated that atorvastatin/metformin combination therapy did not show a better lipid-lowering effect than atorvastatin, which is similar with the recent clinical and preclinical data [48]. The CAMERA study revealed that metformin did not affect the lipid profile in statin-treated patients [49]. Forouzandeh *et al.* confirmed the plasma cholesterol in apoE−/− mice fed a high-fat diet did not affect and found that metformin markedly reduced atherosclerotic plaques [50]. Earlier studies also suggest that an additional anti-atherosclerotic mechanism of metformin when added to atorvastatin, which is independent of the lipid-lowering effect. Study report is the first, to demonstrate that atorvastatin/metformin combination therapy increases the percentage of large HDL sub fraction. Goldberg *et al.* [51] found that metformin could raise the concentrations of large HDL in a clinical trial. The research article also suggested an inverse association of large HDL sub fraction with coronary artery disease, which may involve reverse cholesterol transport (RCT).

4.3 On antidiabetic activity-clinical studies

In a clinical study a great number of patients are selected and treated with metformin–atorvastatin combination tablet administered as a single daily dose [52]. There is only a minor chance for toxic drug interactions when treated with metformin and statin together because metformin is not metabolized and is the mechanism for most statins are via the cytochrome P450 system [53]. Since metformin shows beneficial effects on both dyslipidemia and glycemic control and has been shown to reduce CVD risk while statins may have an added benefi-cial effect on CVD risk. Hence the combined treatment with both drugs seems a good option. Clinical studies on the effects of metformin and statin combination therapy have been carried out but for different diabetic complications [54–56]. Each of these studies had different objectives and included different patients groups, i.e. either with T2DM, dyslipidemia, treated (different doses), untreated, or newly diagnosed T2DM. This criteria were compared in these studies to arrive at overall results of metformin statin combination therapy. The lowest dose of metformin (500 mg) and atorvastatin (10 mg) once daily resulted in the highest reduction of fasting plasma glucose (−35%). Atorvastatin 20 mg showed to attenu-ate the glucose and HbA1c-lowering effect in combination with 1000 and 2000 mg metformin.

In another clinical trial, a total of 50 newly diagnosed patients with T2DM with age range of 47.8 ± 7.4 years and prescribed 850 mg/day of metformin (sustained release), with dietary restriction, were enrolled in open-label multi center pilot study. WHO criteria was followed for the selection of newly diagnosed patients [57] and underwent a physical examination and information about their medical history, demographic parameters, and medication history were obtained by ques-tionnaire. The patients received a constant dose regimen of metformin during the 90-day study period. In that study, the use of metformin in newly diagnosed T2DM patients, improves body weight and glycemic control; however, the addition of low-dose atorvastatin did not improve these conditions. Metformin, in a long-term study, reduces the risk of macrovascular disease after a follow-up period of 4 years [58], and this beneficial effect supports to continue metformin treatment with T2DM patients unless contraindicated. The result of this study is consistent with that reported in an experimental animal model, which indicates that the combination of atorvastatin with metformin did not produce a better lipid-lowering effect than atorvastatin [59]. In addition, the study indicated that 10 mg/day did not increase the HbA1c and serum glucose levels, but there was no additional significant improvement in the studied markers when compared with the metformin-treated group.

4.4 On lipid metabolism -clinical studies

The effects of metformin on lipid homeostasis discussed earlier in this chapter, indicate that lipid metabolism is positively affected in the intestine and liver leading to decreased plasma triglycerides, LDL-C, and total cholesterol. Metformin effects on lipid metabolism seem to be localized to the intestine. Statins mainly act on plasma cholesterol via activation of the LDL-receptor suggesting that combination therapy should show an additional effect on plasma lipids. Combination therapy with statins and metformin demonstrated beneficial effects in patients with other disease(s)/disorder(s) than T2DM and dyslipidemia [60].

In earlier studies, the effect of metformin alone on the lipid profile was studied, and the result analysis showed that only TG levels and LDL/HDL ratio were significantly improved. Whereas these effects were not significantly different compared with its combination with atorvastatin that improves all lipid profile components. These results indicated that the addition of atorvastatin with metformin did not influence the lipid-lowering effects of monotherapy in newly diagnosed T2DM patients with metformin. In previous studies, although metformin moderately improves the lipid profile, there were inconsistencies in its effects on the lipid parameters [61]. Accordingly, the addition of atorvastatin to metformin treatment in newly diagnosed T2DM patients showed relatively normal lipid profile may be irrational and cost ineffective and the emergence of adverse effects may be highly expected with long-term use.

4.5 On prostrate cancer-clinical studies

Diabetic patients receiving metformin have been shown to have a reduced cancer incidence and a decrease in cancer-specific mortality [62]. Statin use was also found to be associated with a reduction in the risk of biochemical recurrence in patients with prostate cancer and a decreased risk of cancer mortality [63, 64]. Based on epidemiologic evidence and the preclinical data for metformin and atorvastatin individually in prostate cancer, the author concluded the beneficial effects of metformin and atorvastatin alone or in combination on SCID mice and cultured prostate cancer cells. Metformin and atorvastatin in combination exhibited potent inhibitory effect on the growth of prostate cancer cells *in vivo* and *in vitro*. The drug combination stimulated apoptosis in prostate cancer cells compared with individual treatment. Mariel concluded that, coupled with epidemiological studies, provide a strong rationale for clinically evaluating the combination of metformin and atorvastatin in prostate cancer patients [17].Recent studies showed that metformin in combination with simvastatin induced G1-phase cell cycle arrest, and Ripk1- and Ripk3-dependent necrosis in prostate cancer cells [65, 66]. The combination of metformin and simvastatin was found to decrease the levels of phospho-Akt and phospho-AMPKα1/α2 [67].

4.6 Combination therapy on other diseases

In T2DM patients with non-alcoholic fatty liver disease (NAFLD) the combination therapy was found to be benefited. Whereas, statin therapy associates negatively with non-alcoholic steatohepatitis and found to be significant fibrosis while a safe use of metformin in patients with T2DM and NAFLD was demonstrated [68]. Combination therapy consisting of metformin and statin treatment is frequently prescribed to women with polycystic ovary syndrome (PCOS). This syndrome increases the risk of T2DM and cardiovascular morbidity as it is associated with abnormal increased lipid levels, insulin resistance, endothelial dysfunction and systemic inflammation [69]. Meta-analysis showed that combined therapy in women with PCOS resulted in improved inflammation and lipid markers but it did not improve insulin sensitivity [70].

Treatments using statins, and combined statins and metformin can effectively improve IR, fasting insulin (F-INS), insulin sensitivity index, hyperandrogenemia, acne, hirsutism, testosterone and decreasing C reactive protein (CRP) [71–73]. Pre-treatment with atorvastatin for 3 months followed by metformin in patients with PCOS improves insulin and homeostasis model assessment of IR (HOMA-IR) indices and reduces CRP level but does not improve the lipid profile compared with placebo treatment. Hence, atorvastatin pre-treatment enhances the effects of metformin in improving IR, whereas inflammatory markers are not affected by decreased total cholesterol (TC) and low-density lipoprotein cholesterol (LDL-C) after cessation of atorvastatin [74].

The lipid-lowering effect of statins administered with or without metformin in PCOS patients remains ambiguous. This finding is also supported with the meta-analysis performed by Gao et al. [75]. A clinical trial demonstrated that insulin secretion was found to be increased after 6 weeks of statin therapy in women with PCOS [76]. The meta-analysis found that statins fail to improve F-INS and HOMA-IR in single or in combination with metformin. This finding may be due to the following reasons. First, statins may damage endothelial function through loss of the protective anti-proliferative and anti-angiogenic effects of adiponectin, resulting in impaired insulin sensitivity [77]. Second, statins decrease the levels of cholesterol mediated by the farnesoid X receptor (FXR), the deficiency of which is related to IR [78]. The activation of FXR can lower the levels of glucose-6-phosphatase, reduce phosphoenol pyruvate carboxykinase in gluconeogenesis, and increase glycogen synthesis [79]. Hence, induced IR caused by statin therapy may be related to the low expression of FXR [80]. Third, statins (lipophilic) are possibly absorbed by extra-hepatic cells; these statins can deregulate cholesterol metabolism, thus deteriorating IR and attenuating β-cell function [81].

Combination therapy could also be considered for T2DM patients with diabetic retinopathy. Diabetic retinopathy (DR) is a microvascular complication of diabetes caused by hyperglycemia and hyperosmolarity. In T2DM patients and pre-existing DR patients, the use of statin showed a protective effect against development of diabetic macular edema [82]. In T2DM patients receiving statin therapy in combination with increased levels of cholesterol remnants and triglycerides were associated with slight decreased in left ventricular systolic function. Targeting cholesterol remnants might be beneficial for finding cardiac function in T2DM patients receiving statins [83].

5. Combination therapy of metformin and simvastatin- clinical studies

A high daily dose of metformin (3000 mg) and simvastatin (40 mg) resulted in an improved insulin resistance, but fasting plasma glucose decreased only by 5%, and observed minor changes on lipid metabolism parameters. This may probably due to the fact that metformin was given on top of simvastatin treatment. The patients involved in these studies had an impaired fasting glucose, dyslipidemia, newly diagnosed T2DM and/or dyslipidemia. However, it could be used for hypothesis-generation rather than making rigid decisions, considering the lack of multiple dose dependent combination studies.

The combination of metformin with insulin may be a better therapeutic option for patients with DM whose hyperglycemia is poorly controlled on insulin treatment. Aviles et al. [84] stated that increased frequency of dosage of insulin causes more improvement in glycemic control and significantly reduce HbA1c which was compared with a combination therapy of insulin and metformin. Furthermore, unchanged FBG and PPBG and HbA1c in patients on metformin and insulin compared to combination of metformin, insulin and simvastatin treated patients. The HbA1c of diabetic patients on simvastatin showed a slight elevation as compared to other groups. Previous studies reported that statin use is associated with a rise of FPG in patients with and without DM [85]. Sattar et al., have identified deterioration in glucose homoeostasis in patients treated with statins and this depends on lipid solubility of statins. Simvastatin can enter easily extra hepatic cells because of its high lipid solubility and may suppress isoprenoid protein synthesis, thus attenuating the action of insulin. The abnormal level of FBG may translate into clinical syndrome of DM with rise in HbA1c is not excluded. The combination of metformin and insulin may be an attractive therapeutic option for patients with DM whose hyperglycemia is poorly controlled on insulin [86].

6. Conclusion

The mechanism of metformin is a controversial along with the use of statins in diabetes. Although the potential detrimental effects of statin therapy on muscle and liver have been known for a long time, new concerns have emerged regarding the risk of new onset diabetes (NOM) that often leads to discontinuation of statin, concerns correlating with initiating statin therapy or non-adherence to therapy.

Metformin is generally to exert its beneficial effects on glucose metabolism mainly in the liver. In line with recent research articles on the topic we conclude that the drug acts primarily in the intestine. This is due to the at least one order of magnitude higher concentrations of metformin in the intestine than in the liver. The drug present in the liver and its effects may be localized to this organ most probably via its effects on gluconeogenesis. A newly diagnosed patient with T2DM who show inadequate response to metformin may need better treatment approaches to lower atherogenic lipids. Supplementation with niacin or high-dose omega-3 fatty acid could be used in newly diagnosed T2DM patients with borderline values of lipid profile, secondary to lifestyle modifications before using a potent statin such as atorvastatin as the first treatment priority.

The effects of metformin on lipid metabolism as discussed in this chapter indicate that lipid level is positively affected in the intestine and liver leading to decreased LDL-C, plasma triglycerides and total cholesterol. Metformin effects on lipid metabolism seem to be localized to the intestine. Statins mainly act on plasma cholesterol levels via activation of the LDL-receptor suggesting that combination therapy should show an additional effect on plasma lipids. This may influence glucose homeostasis primarily by inhibition of insulin secretion in pancreatic β cells. T2DM patients receiving statin therapy in combination, with increased levels of cholesterol remnants and triglycerides were associated with slight decreased in left ventricular systolic function. Targeting cholesterol remnants in addition to T2DM patients receiving statins might be shown beneficial effect on patient's cardiac function. To treat T2DM and its secondary complications, the combination therapy of metformin with statins seems well placed and may act as a double-sided sword particularly in the case of statins. Whereas, statins alone increases the risk on T2DM particularly in pre-diabetic subjects, and co-treatment with metformin might reduce this risk.

We have concluded that, previous studies investigated possible sites of interaction of metformin and statins and they act on largely parallel pathways. Many studies suggested that the benefits of statin therapy for diabetes far outweigh any real or perceived risks, not suggested/recommended for discontinuation of statins for diabetic patients. In conclusion, both metformin and atorvastatin can protect DCM via the mechanism of anti-inflammation and anti-apoptosis activities. The combined administration of metformin and atorvastatin resulted in superior protective effects on DCM than a single drug treatment. In this chapter, we have compiled the possible sites of interaction of metformin and statins and conclude that they act on largely parallel pathways.

Conflict of interest

The authors declare no conflict of interest among themselves.

Abbreviations

BA	bile acids
BMI	body mass index
CVD	cardiovascular disease
DCM	Diabetes cardiomyopathy
DI	disposition indices
DR	diabetic retinopathy
DM	Diabetes mellitus
EGP	endogenous glucose
FBG	Fasting blood glucose
FAS	fatty acid synthase
FFA	free fatty acid
GLUT	glucose transporter
HbA1c	glycated hemoglobin
HDL-C	high-density lipoprotein cholesterol
HMGCR	3-hydroxy-3-methyl-glutaryl-coenzyme A reductase
HMGCS	HMG-CoA synthase
IFG	impaired fasting glucose
IHD	Ischemic heart disease
LDL-C	low-density lipoprotein
NOM	Non onset diabetes
OCT	organic cation transporter
PDX	insulin promoter factor
PMAT	Plasma monoamine transporter
PXR	pregnane X receptor
RCT	Reverse cholesterol transport
RXR	retinoid X receptor
SERT	sodium-dependent serotonin transporter
TNF	Tumor necrosis factor

T2DM	type 2 diabetes mellitus
TG	triglycerides
THTR	thiamine transporter

Author details

Sabu Mandumpal Chacko[1*] and Priya Thambi Thekkekara[2]

1 Mookambika College of Pharmaceutical Sciences and Research, Muvattupuzha, Kerala, India

2 Department of Chemistry, Baselius College, Kottayam, Kerala, India

*Address all correspondence to: mcsabu74@gmail.com

IntechOpen

References

[1] Hu FB. Globalization of diabetes: The role of diet, lifestyle, and genes. Diabetes Care. 2011;**34**(6):1249-1257

[2] World Health Organization. Definition, Diagnosis and Classification of Diabetes Mellitus and its Complications. 1999

[3] Kirpichnikov D, McFarlane SI, Sowers JR. Metformin: An update. Annual International Medicine. 2002; **137**(1):25-33

[4] Miller RA, Chu Q, Xie J. Biguanides suppress hepatic glucagon signalling by decreasing production of cyclic AMP. Nature. 2013;**494**(7436):256-260

[5] Collier CA, Bruce CR, Smith AC. Metformin counters the insulin-induced suppression of fatty acid oxidation and stimulation of triacylglycerol storage in rodent skeletal muscle. American Journal of Physiology Endocrinology Metabolism. 2006;**291**(1):E182-E189

[6] Sherif FM, Ahmed SS. Diabetes and hypertension. International Diabetes Digest. 1997;**8**:1-5

[7] Fischer J, Ganellin CR, Ganesan A, Proudfoot J. Standalone drugs. In: Ganellin JFACR, editor. Analogue-based drug discovery. Weinheim: Wiley-VCH Verlag GmbH & Co; 2010

[8] Timmins P, Donahue S, Meeker J, Marathe P. Steady-state pharmacokinetics of a novel extended-release metformin formulation. Clinical Pharmacokinetics. 2005;**44**(7):721-729

[9] Buse JB, DeFronzo RA, Rosenstock J, Kim T, Burns C, Skare S, et al. The primary glucose-lowering effect of metformin resides in the gut, not the circulation: Results from short-term pharmacokinetic and 12-week dose-ranging studies. Diabetes Care. 2016; **39**(2):198-205

[10] Hashimoto Y, Tanaka M, Okada H, Mistuhashi K, Kimura T, Kitagawa N, et al. Ostprandial hyperglycemia was ameliorated by taking metformin 30 min before a meal than taking metformin with a meal; a randomized, open-label, crossover pilot study. Endocrine. 2016;**52**(2):271-276

[11] Han TK, Proctor WR, Costales CL, Cai H, Everett RS, Thakker DR. Four cation-selective transporters contribute to apical uptake and accumulation of metformin in Caco-2 cell monolayers. The Journal of Pharmacology and Experimental Therapeutics. 2015; **352**(3):519-528

[12] Gormsen LC, Sundelin EI, Jensen JB, Vendelbo MH, Jakobsen S, Munk OL, et al. In vivo imaging of human 11C-metformin in peripheral organs: Dosimetry, biodistribution and kinetic analyses. Journal of Nuclear Medicine. 2016;**57**(12):1920-1926

[13] Bailey CJ, Wilcock C, Scarpello JH. Metformin and the intestine. Diabetologia. 2008;**51**(8):1552-1563

[14] Wilcock C, Wyre ND, Bailey CJ. Subcellular distribution of metformin in rat liver. Journal of Pharmacy and Pharmacology. 1991;**43**(6):442-444

[15] Kinaan M, Ding H, Triggle CR. Metformin: An old drug for the treatment of diabetes but a new drug for the protection of the endothelium. Medicine Principle Practice. 2015; **24**(5):401-415

[16] Bridges HR, Sirvio VA, Agip AN, Hirst J. Molecular features of biguanides required for targeting of mitochondrial respiratory complex I and activation of AMP-kinase. BMC Biology. 2016; **14**:65-70

[17] Chien HC, Zur AA, Maurer TS, Yee SW, Tolsma J, Jasper P, et al. Rapid

method to determine intracellular drug concentrations in cellular uptake assays: Application to metformin in organic cation transporter 1-transfected human embryonic kidney 293 cells. Drug Metabolism Disposal. 2016;**44**(3): 356-364

[18] Gruszka A. New insight into the mechanisms of the anti-hyperglycemic action of metformin. British Journal Medical Research. 2016;**13**:1-9

[19] Chakraborty A, Chowdhury S, Bhattacharyya M. Effect of metformin on oxidative stress, nitrosative stress and inflammatory biomarkers in type 2 diabetes patients. Diabetes Research and Clinical Practice. 2011;**93**(1):56-62

[20] Kashi Z, Mahrooz A, Kianmehr A, Alizadeh A. The role of metformin response in lipid metabolism in patients with recent-onset type 2 diabetes:HbA1c level as a criterion for designating patients as responders or nonresponders to metformin. PLoS One. 2016; **11**(3):e0151543

[21] Zhang C, Gao F, Luo H, Zhang CT, Zhang R. Differential response in levels of high-density lipoprotein cholesterol to one-year metformin treatment in prediabetic patients by race/ethnicity. Cardiovascular Diabetology. 2015;**14**:79

[22] Sonne DP, Knop FK. Comment on Xu et al. Effects of metformin on metabolite profiles and LDL cholesterol in patients with type 2 diabetes. Diabetes Care 2015;38:1858-1867.

[23] Hofmann AF, Hagey LR. Key discoveries in bile acid chemistry and biology and their clinical applications: History of the last eight decades. Journal of Lipid Research. 2014;**55**(8):1553-1595

[24] Wang J, Yang X, Zhang J. Bridges between mitochondrial oxidative stress, ER stress and mTOR signaling in pancreatic β cells. Cell Signaling. 2016; **28**(8):1099-1104

[25] Tanaka K, Saisho Y, Manesso E, Tanaka M, Meguro S, Irie J, et al. Effects of liraglutidemonotherapy onbeta cell function and pancreatic enzymes compared with metforminin Japanese overweight/obese patients with type 2 diabetes mellitus: A subpopulation analysis of the KIND-LM randomized trial. Clinical Drug Investigation. 2015; **35**(10):675-684

[26] Force USPST, Bibbins-Domingo K, Grossman DC, Curry SJ, Davidson KW, Epling JW Jr, et al. Statin use for the primary prevention of cardiovascular disease in adults: US preventive services task force recommendation statement. JAMA. 2016;**316**(19):1997-2007

[27] Gruzdeva O, Uchasova E, Dyleva Y, Akbasheva O, Karetnikova V, Shilov A, et al. Effect of different doses of statins on the development of type 2 diabetes mellitus in patients with myocardial infarction. Diabetes Metabolic Syndrom Obesity Targets and Therapetics. 2017; **10**:481-490

[28] Gruzdeva O, Uchasova E, Dyleva Y, Akbasheva O, Karetnikova V, Barbarash O. Early effects of treatment low-dose atorvastatin on markers of insulin resistance and inflammation in patients with myocardial infarction. Frontrier Pharmacology. 2016;**7**:324-330

[29] Wang S, Cai R, Yuan Y, Varghese Z, Moorhead J, Ruan XZ. Association between reductions in low-density lipoprotein cholesterol with statin therapy and the risk of new-onset diabetes: A meta-analysis. Science Reports. 2017;**7**:39982

[30] Ruscica M, Macchi C, Morlotti B, Sirtori CR, Magni P. Statin therapy and related risk of new-onset type 2 diabetes mellitus. European Journal of International Medicine. 2014;**25**(5): 401-406

[31] Hao M, Head WS, Gunawardana SC, Hasty AH, Piston DW. Direct effect of

cholesterol on insulin secretion: A novel mechanism for pancreatic beta-cell dysfunction. Diabetes. 2007;**56**(9): 2328-2338

[32] Zhou J, Li W, Xie Q, Hou Y, Zhan S, Yang X, et al. Effects of simvastatin on glucose metabolism in mouse MIN6 cells. Journal Diabetes Research. 2014; **2014**:376570

[33] Scattolini V, Luni C, Zambon A, Galvanin S, Gagliano O, Ciubotaru CD, et al. Simvastatin rapidly and reversibly inhibits insulin secretion in intact single-islet cultures. Diabetes Therapetics. 2016;**7**(4):679-693

[34] Nakata M, Nagasaka S, Kusaka I, Matsuoka H, Ishibashi S, Yada T. Effects of statins on the adipocyte maturation and expression of glucose transporter 4 (SLC2A4): Implications in glycaemic control. Diabetologia. 2006;**49**(8): 1881-1892

[35] Nicolucci A. Epidemiological aspects of neoplasms in diabetes. ActaDiabetologica. 2010;**47**(2):87-95

[36] Ma RCW, Chan JCN. Type 2 diabetes in East Asians: Similarities and differences with populations in Europe and the United States. Annals of the New York Academy of Sciences. 2013; **1281**(1):64-91

[37] LashTL RAH, OstenfeldEB. Associations of statin use with colorectal cancer recurrence and mortality in a Danish cohort. American Journal of Epidemiology. 2017;**186**(6): 679-687

[38] He Y, Huang H, Farischon C. Combined effects of atorvastatin and aspirin on growth and apoptosis in human prostate cancer cells. Oncology Reports. 2017;**37**(2):953-960

[39] Oliveira KA, Dal-Cim T, Lopes FG, Ludka FK, Nedel CB, Tasca CI. Atorvastatin promotes cytotoxicity and

reduces migration and proliferation of human A172 glioma cells. Molecular Neurobiology. 2018;**55**(2):1509-1523

[40] Tapia-Pérez JH, Preininger R, Kirches E. Simultaneous administration of statins and pioglitazone limits tumorgrowth in a rat model of malignant glioma. Anticancer Research. 2016;**36**(12):6357-6366

[41] Fei L, Yuan G, Gui-yun R, Jun-ke L, Xi-long Z, Qin Z, et al. Combined use of metformin and atorvastatin attenuates atherosclerosis in rabbits fed a high-cholesterol diet. Scientific Reports. 2017;**7**:1-10

[42] Islam M, Alam A, Rahman M, Ali Y, Mamun A, Rahman M, et al. Effects of combination of antidiabetic agent and statin on alloxan-induced diabetes with cardiovascular diseases in rats. Journal of Scientific Research. 2012;**4**(3): 709-720

[43] Matafome P, Louro T, Rodrigues L, Crisostomo J, Nunes E, Amaral C, et al. Metformin and atorvastatin combination further protect the liver in type 2 diabetes with hyperlipidaemia. Diabetes/Metabolism Research and Reviews. 2011;**27**(1):54-62

[44] Luo B, Li B, Wang W, Liu X, Liu X, Xia Y. Rosuvastatin alleviates diabetic cardiomyopathy by inhibiting NLRP3 inflammation and MAPK pathways in a type 2 diabetes rat model. Cardiovascular Drugs and Therapy. 2014;**28**:33-43

[45] Weikun J, Tao B, Jiang Z, Zijing N, Daogui F, Xin X, et al. Combined administration of metformin and atorvastatin attenuates diabetic cardiomyopathy by inhibiting inflammation, apoptosis, and oxidative stress in type 2 diabetic mice. Cell and developmental Biology. 2021;**9**:1-14

[46] Li Y. Urotensin II promotes atherosclerosis in cholesterol-fed rabbits. PLoS One. 2014;**9**:57-64

[47] Mora S. Lipoprotein particle profiles by nuclear magnetic resonance compared with standard lipids and apolipoproteins in predicting incident cardiovascular disease in women. Circulation. 2009;**119**:931-939

[48] Kooy A. Long-term effects of metformin on metabolism and microvascular and macrovascular disease in patients with type 2 diabetes mellitus. Archives of Internal Medicine. 2009;**169**:616-625

[49] Preiss D. Metformin for non-diabetic patients with coronary heart disease (the CAMERA study): A randomised controlled trial. The Lancet. Diabetes & Endocrinology. 2014;**2**:116-124

[50] Forouzandeh F. Metformin beyond diabetes: Pleiotropic benefits of metformin in attenuation of atherosclerosis. Journal of the American Heart Association. 2014;**3**:8-15

[51] Goldberg R. Lifestyle and metformin treatment favorably influence lipoprotein subfraction distribution in the Diabetes Prevention Program. The Journal of Clinical Endocrinology and Metabolism. 2013;**98**:3989-3998

[52] Oh JH, Eun Lee J, Jeong Kim Y, Oh TO, Han S, Jeon EK, et al. Designing of the fixed-dose gastroretentive bilayer tablet for sustained release of metformin and immediate release of atorvastatin. Drug Delivery Indian Pharmacy. 2016;**42**(2):340-349

[53] Scheen AJ. Drug interactions of clinical importance with antihyperglycaemic agents: An update. Drug Safety. 2005;**28**(7):601-631

[54] Krysiak R, Okopien B. Haemostatic effects of metformin in simvastatin treated volunteers with impaired fasting glucose. Basic & Clinical Pharmacology & Toxicology. 2012;**111**(6):380-384

[55] Krysiak R, Okopien B. The effect of metformin on monocyte secretory function in simvastatin-treated patients with impaired fasting glucose. Metabolism. 2013;**62**(1):39-43

[56] Hao Z, Liu Y, Liao H, Zheng D, Xiao C, Li G. Atorvastatin plus metformin confer additive benefits on subjects with dyslipidemia and overweight/ obese via reducing ROCK2 concentration. Experimental and Clinical Endocrinology & Diabetes. 2016;**124**(4):246-250

[57] Bennet PH. Impact of the new WHO classification and diagnostic criteria. Diabetes, Obesity & Metabolism. 1999;**1**(1):1-6

[58] Kooy A, de Jager J, Lehert P, Bets D, Wulffelé MG, Donker AJ. Long-term effects of metformin on metabolism and microvascular and macrovascular disease in patients with Type 2 diabetes mellitus. Archives of Internal Medicine. 2009;**169**:616-625

[59] Luo F, Guo Y, Ruan GY, Long JK, Zheng XL, Xia Q. Combined use of metformin and atorvastatin attenuates atherosclerosis in rabbits fed a high-cholesterol diet. Science Reporter. 2017;7:2169

[60] Khan TJ, Ahmed YM, Zamzami MA, Siddiqui AM, Khan I, Baothman OAS, et al. Atorvastatin treatment modulates the gut microbiota of the hypercholesterolemic patients. OMICS. 2018;**22**(2):154-163

[61] Buse JB, Tan MH, Prince MJ, Erickson PP. The effects of oral anti-hyperglycemic medications on serum lipid profiles in patients with Type 2 diabetes. Diabetes Obesity. Metabolism. 2004;**6**:133-156

[62] DeCensi A, Puntoni M, Goodwin P, Cazzaniga M, Gennari A, Bonanni B, et al. Metformin and cancer risk in diabetic patients:a systematic review

and meta-analysis. Cancer Prevention Research. 2010;**3**:1451-1461

[63] Allott EH, Howard LE, Cooperberg MR, Kane CJ, Aronson WJ, Terris MK, et al. Postoperative statin use and risk of biochemical recurrence following radical prostatectomy: Results from the Shared Equal Access Regional Cancer Hospital (SEARCH) database. BJU International. 2014;**114**:661-666

[64] Yu O, Eberg M, Benayoun S, Aprikian A, Batist G, Suissa S, et al. Use of statins and the risk of death in patients with prostate cancer. Journal of Clinical Oncology. 2014;**32**:5-11

[65] Pennanen P, Syvälä H, Bläuer M, Savinainen K, Ylikomi T, Tammela TL, et al. The effects of metformin and simvastatin onthe growth of LNCaP and RWPE-1 prostate epithelial cell lines. European Journal of Pharmacology. 2016;**788**:160-167

[66] Babcook MA, Sramkoski RM, Fujioka H, Daneshgari F, Almasan A, Shukla S, et al. Combination simvastatin and metformin induces G1-phase cell cycle arrest and Ripk1- and Ripk3-dependent necrosis in C4-2B osseous metastatic castration resistant prostate cancer cells. Cell Death & Disease. 2014;**5**:1536

[67] Babcook MA, Shukla S, Fu P, Vazquez EJ, Puchowicz MA, Molter JP, et al. Synergistic simvastatin and metformin combination chemotherapy for osseous metastatic castration-resistant prostate cancer. Molecular Cancer Therapeutics. 2014;**13**: 2288-2302

[68] Nascimbeni F, Aron-Wisnewsky J, Pais R, Tordjman J, Poitou C, Charlotte F, et al. Statins, antidiabetic medications and liver histology in patients with diabetes with non-alcoholic fatty liver disease. BMJ Open Gastroenterology. 2016;**3**(1):e000075

[69] Ehrmann DA. Polycystic ovary syndrome. The New England Journal of Medicine. 2005;**352**(12):1223-1236

[70] Sun J, Yuan Y, Cai R, Sun H, Zhou Y, Wang P, et al. An investigation into the therapeutic effects of statins with metformin on polycystic ovary syndrome: A meta-analysis of randomised controlled trials. BMJ Open. 2015;**5**(3):e007280

[71] Kazerooni T, Shojaei-Baghini A, Dehbashi S, et al. Effects of metformin plus simvastatin on polycystic ovary syndrome: Aprospective, randomized, double-blind, placebo-controlled study. FertilSteril. 2010;**94**:2208-2213

[72] Banaszewska B, Pawelczyk L, Spaczynski RZ. Effects of simvastatin and metformin on polycystic ovary syndrome after sixmonths of treatment. Journal of Clinical Endocrinology and Metabolism. 2011;**96**:3493-3501

[73] Banaszewska B, Pawelczyk L, Spaczynski RZ. Comparison of simvastatin and metformin in treatment of polycystic ovary syndrome: Prospective randomized trial. Journal of Clinical Endocrinology and Metabolism. 2009;**94**:4938-4945

[74] Sathyapalan T, Kilpatrick ES, Coady AM. Atorvastatin pretreatment augments the effect of metformin in patients with polycystic ovary syndrome (PCOS). Clinical Endocrinology. 2010; **72**:566-568

[75] Gao L, Zhao FL, Li SC. Statin is a reasonable treatment option for patients with polycystic ovary syndrome: A meta-analysis of randomized controlled trials. Experimental and Clinical Endocrinology & Diabetes. 2012; **120**:367-375

[76] Raja-Khan N, Kunselman AR, Hogeman CS. Effects of atorvastatin on vascular function, inflammation, and androgens in women with polycystic

ovary syndrome: A double-blind, randomized, placebo-controlled trial. Fertility and Sterility. 2011;**95**: 1849-1852

[77] Rocco MB. Statins and diabetes risk: Fact, fiction, and clinical implications. Cleveland Clinic Journal of Medicine. 2012;**79**:883-893

[78] Cariou B, Nan Harmelen K, Duran-Sandoval D. The farnesoid X receptor modulates adiposity and peripheral insulin sensitivity in mice. Journal of Biological Chemistry. 2006;**281**:11039-11049

[79] Kobayashi M, Ikegami H, Fujisawa T. Prevention and treatment of obesity, insulin resistance, and diabetes by bile acid-binding resin. Diabetes. 2007;**56**:239-247

[80] Wang L, Huang X, Hu S, et al. Effect of simvastatin on the expression of farnesoid X receptor in diabetic animal models of altered glucose homeostasis. Chinese Medicinal Journal (Engl). 2014;**127**:218-224

[81] Koh KK, Quon MJ, Han SH, et al. Differential metabolic effects of pravastatin and simvastatin in hypercholesterolemic patients. Atherosclerosis. 2009;**204**:483-490

[82] Chung Y-R, Park SW, Choi S-Y, Kim SW, Moon KY, Kim JH, et al. Association of statin use and hypertriglyceridemia with diabetic macular edema in patients with type 2 diabetes and diabetic retinopathy. Cardiovascular Diabetology. 2017; **16**(1):4

[83] Jorgensen PG, Jensen MT, Biering-Sorensen T, Mogelvang R, Galatius S, Fritz-Hansen T, et al. Cholesterol remnants and triglycerides are associated with decreased myocardial function in patients with type 2 diabetes. Cardiovascular Diabetology. 2016;**15**(1):137

[84] Aviles-Santa L, Sinding J, Raskin P. Effects of metformin in patients with poorly controlled insulin-treated type 2 diabetes mellitus. Annual Internal Medicine. 1999;**131**(3):182-188

[85] Sukhija R, Prayaga S, Marashdeh M. Effect of statins on fasting plasma glucose in diabetic and nondiabetic patients. Journal of Investigational Medicine. 2009;**57**(3):495-499

[86] Sattar N, Preiss D, Murray HM. Statins and risk of incident diabetes: A collaborative meta-analysis of randomized statin trials. Lancet. 2010;**375**(9716):735-742

Section 4

Metformin and
Tuberculosis

Chapter 7

Metformin for Tuberculosis Infection

Bernadette Dian Novita, Ari Christy Mulyono and Ferdinand Erwin

Abstract

Tuberculosis, caused by *Mycobacterium tuberculosis* (M.tb), remains the biggest infection burden in the word. Rifampin (RIF) and Isoniazid (INH) are the most effective antibiotics for killing M.tb. However, the resistance rate of rifampin and INH are high and lead to almost 35% treatment failure. Metformin enhanced anti tuberculosis efficacy in killing *M. tuberculosis* through several mechanism, firstly through autophagia mechanism and secondly by activating superoxide dismutase (SOD). Metformin activated mTOR and AMPK then induced more effective autophagy against M.tb. Superoxide Dismutase (SOD) is an enzyme produced in the host's antioxidant defense system. SOD neutralizes reactive oxygen species (ROS) that excessively produced during phagocytosis process against M.tb. Excessive production of ROS associated with Th1 overactivation and leads into macrophage activity inhibition and excessive tissue damage. Metformin has ability in improving SOD level during inflammation.

Keywords: metformin, tuberculosis, autophagia, anti tuberculosis enhancement

1. Introduction

Metformin is a biguanide salt hydrochloride consists of a molecular component of $C_4H_{11}N_5$.HCl (*N,N*-Dimethyl imido dicarboximide diamide). Metformin is unmetabolized and widely distributed to all body tissues including the intestine, liver and kidney. Metformin is also excreted unchanged [1, 2]. Metformin undergoes a methylation process binds to the monoamine transporter called organic cation transporter group (SLC 29A4/SLC 22A1/SLC 47A1), then plays a role in the redox reaction of the DNA synthesis process and stimulates AMPK through inhibition of the mitochondrial complex I reaction and activation of mitochondrial reactive nitrogen species (RNS) and phosphoinoside-3-kinase (PI3K) [2].

Metformin use oral anti-diabetic in type-2 DM patients for almost a decade [3], works through AMPK activation, thus increase insulin receptor sensitivity. AMPK activation also inhibits hepatic gluconeogenesis and glycogenolysis process and then glucose uptake may increase. This process may lead the increase of lactic acid production, especially when anaerobic glucose metabolism occurs. In addition, metformin effectively increase insulin activity in the musculoskeletal and liver by doing exercising or active physical activity thereby increasing energy requirements and metabolic responses throughout the body (**Figure 1**).

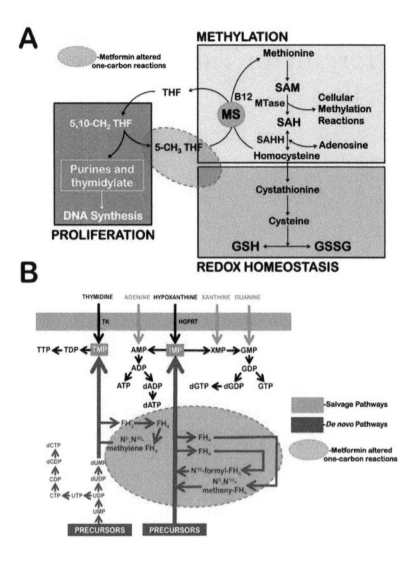

Figure 1.
Methylation process of Metformin in Krebs' cycle [4].

Since, metformin inhibits hepatic gluconeogenesis process, it also reduces metabolic acids flux thus lactic acid accumulated and may lead to metformin associated lactic acidosis (MALA) [5] as seen in **Figure 2**. However, MALA is rarely happened [3, 7].

Indications of metformin treatment in Type 2 DM patients is HbA1C levels within range of 7–8%. Moreover, metformin also use to improve insulin receptor resistance through the AMPK pathway in pre-diabetes type 2 patients with impaired glucose tolerance, obese patients and polycystic ovaries. Contra indication of metformin use: pregnancy and breastfeed, renal insufficiency, liver failure, heart failure lactic acidosis, severe infection, dehydration and alcoholism.

Metformin is excreted by the kidneys in an unchanged form, thus patient with renal dysfunction need to be carefully given [8]. Some studies suggested metformin may still be given to patients with impaired renal function and does not require a dose adjustment whenever the GFR is>40% [9, 10].

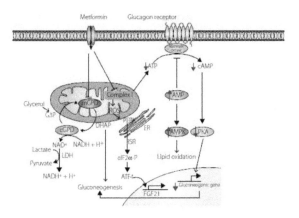

Figure 2.
AMPK stimulation pathway by metformin [6].

2. Tuberculosis, its therapy and resistance mechanism

Tuberculosis (TB) is a chronic infection caused by *Mycobacterium tuberculosis* (Mtb). Tuberculosis remains one of "global health emergency" diseases [11]. Nowadays, the evidence of TB new cases are increasing and some studies said that this situation were associated with the rising number of patients with immunocompromised condition such patients with HIV, diabetes mellitus (DM), cancer and autoimmune diseases [12, 13]. The risk of TB infection in DM patients increased 2,39 times. Moreover, the risk of failure of anti-TB therapy in DM patients also increased 1.69 times [14, 15].

Tuberculosis continues to be difficult to treat, mainly due to three natural barriers: 1) **Cell wall.** *M. tuberculosis* (M.tb) has a waxy appearance, which is due to the composition of the cell walls. More than 60% of the cell wall is lipid, mainly mycolic acids. This extraordinary membrane of M.tb obviates many pharmacological compounds from penetrating the cell membrane or getting inside the cytosol; 2) **Efflux pumps.** The second layer of M.tb defense is provided by the ability of efflux pumps in the cell membrane. Potentially harmful chemicals are pumped out from the bacterial cytoplasm into the extracellular space by these transport proteins. This process contributes to the resistance of mycobacteria to anti-tuberculosis standard; 3) **Location in host.** A third barrier is the propensity of some of the bacilli to hide inside the patient's cells, thereby surrounding themselves with an extra physico-chemical barrier that antimicrobial agents must cross to be effective [2, 16].

First-line anti-TB regiments are rifampicin, isoniazid (INH), ethambutol, pyrazinamide, use as anti-TB. Second line of anti-TB are fluoroquinolone (ciprofloxacin, ofloxacin, levofloxacin, moxifloxacin), ethionamide, PAS, cyclomerize, amikacin, kanamycin, dan capreomycin [2]. Herewith, we discussed more in First-line anti-TB.

Rifampicin are macrocyclic antibiotics. Rifampin or rifampicin, rifapentine, and rifabutin are macrocyclic antibiotics important in the treatment of mycobacterial diseases. Rifampicin binds to the β subunit of DNA-dependent RNA polymerase (*rpoB*) to form a stable drug-enzyme complex, then suppresses chain formation in RNA synthesis [2]. Rifampicin should be taken on an empty stomach, whereas rifapentine should be taken with food if possible. Rifampicin is mostly well tolerated in patients. Less than 4% of patients with TB developing significant adverse reactions; the most common are rash (0.8%), fever (0.5%), and nausea and vomiting (1.5%). Rifampicin is a hepatotoxic agent, however, rarely, hepatitis and deaths due to liver failure in whom had pre-existing liver disease. Chronic liver disease, alcoholism, and old age appear to increase the incidence of severe hepatic problems. GI disturbances have occasionally required discontinuation of the drug. Rifampicin potently induces CYPs 1A2, 2C9, 2C19, and 3A4, and it decreases the $t1/2$ of zid-ovudine, prednisone, digitoxin, quinidine, ketoconazole, propranolol, phenytoin, sulfonylureas, hormonal contraceptive and warfarin [1, 2].

Isoniazid (*isoni*cotinic acid hydr*azide*), also called INH is an important drug for the chemotherapy of drug-susceptible TB. INH enters M.tb membrane cell by passive diffusion. INH is not directly toxic to the bacillus, it must be activated into toxic form for M.tb by KatG, a multifunctional catalase-peroxidase. INH active metabolite, isonicotinoyl, was the product of KatG catalysation. Isonicotinyl interacts with M.tb's NAD and NAPD then produce toxin. The nicotinoyl-NAD isomer, inhibits the activities of enoyl acyl carrier protein reductase (InhA) and KasA. Inhibition of InhA and KasA inhibits synthesis of mycolic acid of the mycobacterial cell wall and then leads to bacterial cell death. A nicotinoyl-NADP isomer, another toxic product of isonicotinyl-NAD and NAPD interaction, inhibits ($Ki < 1$ nM) M.tb dihydrofolate reductase, then interfers nucleic acid synthesis. KatG activation of INH also produce superoxide, H2O2, alkyl hydroperoxides, and the NO radical. These products may also contribute to the INH's mycobactericidal effects, due to the defect od M.tb in the central regulator of the oxidative stress response, *oxyR*. Backup defense against radicals is provided by alkyl hydroperoxide reductase (encoded by *ahpC*), which detoxifies organic peroxides. Increased expression of *ahpC* reduces isoniazid effectiveness [2].

Isoniazid is metabolized by hepatic arylamine NAT2. The patients' clearance of INH classifies into three phenotypic groups: fast, intermediate, and slow acetylators. These acetylator groups relates to NAT2 genotype and influenced by race, not by sex or age. Fast acetylation is found in Inuit and Japanese, while slow acetylation is the predominant phenotype in most Scandinavians, Jews, and North African whites [2]. The high acetyltransferase activity (fast acetylation) relates to high dose demand of INH. After NAT2 converts isoniazid to acetyl isoniazid, which is excreted by the kidney, acetyl isoniazid can also be converted to acetyl hydrazine and then to hepatotoxic metabolites by CYP2E1. Drug-Induced Hepatitis (DIH) associated INH occurs ~0.1% of all patients taking INH. Hepatic damage incidence increases with age but is rare in patients less than 20 years old. The risk is increased ~3% by coadministration INH with rifampicin. Most cases of DIH occur 4–8 weeks after initiation of anti TB therapy [2, 17]. Neuropathy, such as peripheral neuritis (most commonly paraesthesia of feet and hands) is more frequent in slow acetylators and in individuals with diabetes mellitus, poor nutrition, or anemia. To prevent neuropathy, pyridoxine is needed. Isoniazid may also induce syndrome resembling systemic lupus erythematosus. Isoniazid is a potent inhibitor of CYP2C19 and CYP3A and a weak inhibitor of CYP2D6. However, isoniazid induces CYP2E1. Herewith drugs that are metabolized by these enzymes will potentially be affected (**Table 1**) [1, 2].

Pyrazinamide is the synthetic pyrazine analogue of nicotinamide and activated by acidic conditions. Pyrazinamide as anti TB has several mechanisms of action. Pyrazinamide passively diffuses into M.tb cells, and then pyrazinamidase (encoded by the *pncA* gene) deaminates pyrazinamide to pyrazinoic acid (POA−, in its dissociated form). Pyrazinoic acid passively diffuses to POA− to the extracellular milieu. In an acidic extracellular milieu, a fraction of POA− is protonated to the uncharged form, POAH, a more lipid-soluble form. The POAH re-enters back to M.tb cells and accumulates due to a deficient efflux pump [2, 18]. The acidification of the intracellular milieu is believed to inhibit enzyme function and collapse the transmembrane proton motive force, thereby killing the bacteria. Inhibitors of

No	Coadministration Drug	CYP isoform	Adverse Effects
1.	Acetaminophen	CYP2E1 induction	Hepatotoxicity
2.	Carbamazepine	CYP3A inhibition	Neurological toxicity
3.	Diazepam	CYP3A and CYP2C19 inhibition	Sedation and respiratory depression
4.	Ethosuximide	CYP3A inhibition	Psychotic behaviors
5.	Isoflurane and enflurane	CYP2C19 inhibition	Decreased effectiveness of INH
6.	Phenytoin	CYP2C19 inhibition	Neurological toxicity
7.	Theophylline	CYP3A inhibition	Seizures, palpitation, nausea
8.	Vincristine	CYP3A inhibition	Limb weakness and tingling
9.	Warfarin	CYP2C9 inhibition	Bleeding (higher risk with INH doses >300 mg/d

Table 1.
Drugs interact with Isoniazid [2].

energy metabolism or reduced energy production states lead to enhanced pyrazinamide effect. A specific target of pyrazinamide has been proposed to be ribosomal protein S1 (encoded by *RpsA*) in the trans-translation process, so that toxic proteins due to stress accumulate and kill the bacteria. In addition, pyrazinamide's target may include an aspartate decarboxylase (encoded by *panD*) involved in making precursors needed for pantothenate and CoA biosynthesis in persistent Mtb Injury to the liver is the most serious side effect of pyrazinamide. Therefore, all patients should undergo examination of hepatic function prior to pyrazinamide administration to prevent drug-induced hepatitis, and should be repeated at frequent intervals during the entire period of treatment. If evidence of significant hepatic damage becomes apparent, therapy must be stopped. In an individual with hepatic dysfunction, pyrazinamide should not be given unless this is absolutely unavoidable. Pyrazinamide inhibits excretion of urate in nearly all patients, which may cause acute episodes of gout due to hyperuricemia comdition. Other untoward effects observed with pyrazinamide include arthralgias, anorexia, nausea and vomiting, dysuria, malaise, and fever. Because of insufficient data on teratogenicity, the use of pyrazinamide is not approved during pregnancy in the U.S. [1, 2].

Ethambutol hydrochloride is a water-soluble and heat-stable compound. Ethambutol inhibits arabinosyl transferase III, thereby disrupting the transfer of arabinose into arabinogalactan biosynthesis, which in turn disrupts the assembly of mycobacterial cell wall. The arabinosyl transferases are encoded by *embAB* genes. The oral bioavailability of ethambutol is about 80%. Approximately 10–40% of the drug is bound to plasma protein. The decline in ethambutol is biexponential, with a $t1/2$ of 3 h in the first 12 h and a $t1/2$ of 9 h between 12 and 24 h due to redistribution of drug. Clearance and Vd are greater in children than in adults on a per kilogram basis. Slow and incomplete absorption is common in children, so that good peak concentrations of drug are often not achieved with standard dosing. About 80% of the drug is not metabolized at all and is renally excreted. Therefore, in renal failure even in patients receiving hemodialysis, ethambutol does not need dose adjustment. Ethambutol induces very few serious unfavorable reactions: About 1% experience diminished visual acuity, 0.5% a rash, and 0.3% drug fever. Other side effects that have been observed are pruritus, joint pain, malaise, GI upset, abdominal pain, dizziness, headache, disorientation, mental confusion, and possible hallucinations. The most important side effect is optic neuritis, resulting in decreased visual acuity and loss of red-green discrimination. Therefore, ethambutol should not be given in children and pregnancy.

The aim of combination anti TB are 1) increasing bactericidal activity from the very beginning of therapy and 2) preventing pathogen resistance, therefore, patients could be cured. Prevent to death, prevent to recurrence, and cutting off the transmission chains by eradicated Mtb [8, 19]. Rifampicin and isoniazid have the highest bactericidal activity against Mtb, compared to other anti-TB. However, rifampicin and isoniazid are also easily becoming resistance.

Herewith some mechanism of anti-TB resistance: 1) Anti-TB amenable to penetrate into Mtb wall's cell, due to its rich of lipopolysaccharide and mannose; 2) Mtb becomes dormant easily in anaerobic, thus anti-TB, except rifampicin and fluoroquinolone, which aims to inhibit metabolic processes became ineffective in dormant conditions; 3) Alteration of the enzymes that responsible for activating pro-drugs (pyrazinamide and isoniazid); 4) DNA of Mtb mutases; 5) Target protein's structure alters thus the efficacy of rifampicin, ethambutol, streptomycin, fluoroquinolone and macrolide declined (**Figure 3**).

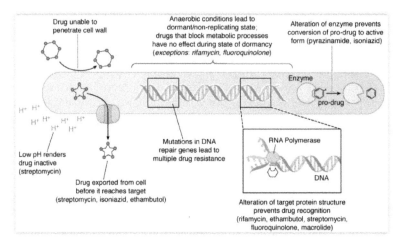

Figure 3.
Anti-TB resistance mechanism against Mtb [2].

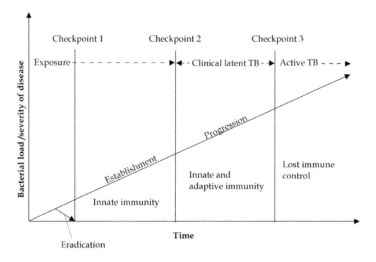

Figure 4.
Escape mechanism of Mtb [20].

Based on in vitro studies, Rifampicin inhibits Mtb at a concentration of 0.06–0.25 mg/L. The prevalence of rifampicin resistance isolates (1 in every 10^7 to 10^8 CFU bacilli). Pyrazinamide has antimicrobial activity in vitro at an acidic pH of 5.8–5.95 and 80–90% of clinical isolates have an MIC (minimum inhibitory concentration) of 100 mg/L. Pyrazinamide resistance occurs due to single point mutations (pncA gene). The minimum inhibitory concentration (MIC) of isoniazid is 0.025–0.05 mg/L. The prevalence of isoniazid resistance occurs at 1 in every 10^6 CFU bacilli. The inhibition of ethambutol is 0.5–2 mg/L and resistance occurs due to the embB gene mutase. Based on this, to prevent anti-TB resistance, it is given in combination [2].

Despite of those anti-TB resistance, Mtb also has ability to manipulate host immune response, both innate and adaptive immune systems or known with escape mechanism (**Figure 4**). Mtb has ability to avoid intracellular killing inside macrophages (phagocytosis) [20].

3. Immune response against *Mycobacterium tuberculosis*

Several epidemiological models of family members who have long shared the bedroom with subjects with TB infection have clearly demonstrated that 5 to 20% of them do not get infected (resilient individuals or resisters), or become transiently infected (early sterilization or early clearance) [21]. An individual defined as resilient after close and prolonged contact with the negativity both of the skin reactivity test and of the IFN-g release assay (IGRA) which persists for at least 1 year. On the other side, the study of TB susceptibility, has reported onto various components of human immunity to mycobacteria. Different genetic polymorphisms which modulate the host immune response in favor of TB infection and disease progression have been identified in human leukocyte antigens (HLA), toll like receptors (TLR), vitamin D receptors (VDR), cytokines with their receptors and many other functional immune components [21].

Transcriptomic studies have described a TB signature of neutrophil-driven IFN-inducible genes in Mtb, including IFN-g but also type I IFNs, reflecting disease extension and response to treatment and highlighting the previously under-appreciated role of IFN-ab signaling in TB pathogenesis. Beyond host factors, bacterial virulence constitutes the other major player when evaluating the risk of TB infection. Differential Mtb gene expression in the different phases of infection also contributes to the bacterial virulence besides bacterial strain or burden in respiratory secretion. Mtb lacks virulence factors such as toxins, and its immune-escaping ability depends on the alteration of lipid metabolism, metal-transporter proteins, and protease, which inhibit the antimicrobial effectors of macrophages [22].

Macrophages are the first line of immune defense, so they can prevent the infection but only if the ratio of forces lies clearly to their advantage [23]. Otherwise, they favor its development because they become first a niche for the slow replication of the Mtb and then the sanctuary for the persistence of the infection inside the phagosome during the latent infection phase. Mtb expresses an extremely wide variety of virulence factors that counteract macrophage ability in suppressing the pathogen. Among Mtb strategies we can include the intracellular trafficking inhibition, autophagy inhibition, cytosol entry ability, the induction of host cell death and the neutralization of toxic components as reactive oxygen species [15, 21].

Whilst IFN-γ is a key element in the containment of Mtb within the Macrophage, it is now widely recognized that performing this function requires the presence of vitamin D. IFN-γ axis is struggling against the ESX-system to enhance phagolysosome activity, vitamin D deficiency abets the Mtb replication [21]. IFN-γ is the chief cytokine involved in the protective immune response against mycobacterial infection [24–26]. The main function of IFN-γ is macrophage activation, thus in this study autophagy marker was also high [27], it referred to its mycobactericidal functions. Predominantly IFN-γ is also contributed to less severe forms of pulmonary TB [28]. Moreover, IFN-γ also enhances the antigen presentation through the induction of the expression of molecules from the major histocompatibility complex (MHC) class I and II and promoting the differentiation of CD4 T lymphocytes to the Th1 subpopulation [26, 29]. Furthermore as conclusion, MET through mTOR inhibition enhances macrophage's autophagy activity thus Th1-related IFN-γ activity increases and in this study, DM-TB coinfection patients represented by BTA conversion. However, IFN-γ relates to CD8 T lymphocytes or cytotoxic T-cells activity which contributes to lung tissue damaged, thus IFN-γ activity needs to be controlled [28, 29].

IL-10 is produced by macrophages and Th-2 during *M. tuberculosis* infection. IL-10, through SOCS 3 activation, acts inhibiting target cells of inflammation, then the production of pro-inflammatory cytokines (IFN-γ,TNF- α and IL-12) reduced [24, 25, 28]. Due to its ability to inhibit the production of pro-inflammatory cytokines, IL-10 has an immune-regulatory function which plays an important role in adequate balancing between inflammatory and immune-pathological responses. However, the increase in IL-10 levels appears to support the mycobacterial survival in the host [28]. IL-10 reduces the protective response to *M. tuberculosis* by inhibiting autophagy targeting signals through IL-10 activated SOCS3, and then, SOCS3 inhibits the Janus kinase-2 (Jak2)/signal transducer and activator of transcription (Stat) pathway in activating macrophage autophagy [24, 25]. In this study, the increasing of IL-10 not only due to macrophage related Th-2 activation, it was insulin attenuated anti-inflammation regulatory. In this study, insulin was used for patients 'hyperglycemic condition [30, 31].

Nitric oxide (NO) within macrophages play less important role in human. On the other hand, reactive oxygen species (ROS) play a well-documented role in the immune response to Mtb, which increases susceptibility in patients displaying mutations in a catalytic subunit of NADPH-oxidase 2 involved in ROS production on phagolysosome membrane. Mtb affects NADPH- oxidase activity through nucleoside diphosphate kinase (Npk) interaction with small GTPases involved in NADPH-oxidase assembly and functioning [21, 32].

Dendritic cells (DCs) play a fundamental role in the immune defense system due to antigen presentation, co- stimulating activity and the large cytokine production capacity with activity on the lymphocytes cluster of differentiation (CD) 4. DCs role in immune response against TB remains controversial. DCs soon become a niche for the Mtb. CD209, also called DC- specific intercellular adhesion molecule 3-grabbing non-integrin receptor (DC-SIGN), represents the gateway of Mtb into the DC [33].

The T lymphocytes immune response begins when Mtb spreads inside the lymph nodes, but its arousal lies in the early activation of the innate immune system. Inside the lymph nodes, T lymphocytes undergo a process of activation and expansion of the specific populations for the Mtb antigens. However, at this point, the largest part is done and the infection is now established. The development of a hypersensitivity response (delayed-type) to intradermal injected tuberculin (DHT) or purified protein derivative indicates cellular immune response in 2–6 weeks after Mtb infection. It is important to underline that DHT positivity does not correlate with protective response to TB, and the disease can occur in people with adequate DHT response [34, 35].

The process of maturation of the phagosome of macrophages is facilitated and increased by IFN-γ, the production of which is mostly dependent on the T lymphocytes CD4+ with a minor support of lymphocytes CD8+ and T lymphocytes with γδ receptor. However, IFN-γ is inadequate to control the infection alone, and it requires the association of other molecules such as IL-6, IL-1, and TNF-α. It is known that TNF-α boosts the production of NO by macrophages and stimulates the production of the chemokines CCL5, CCL9, CXCL10, and CCL2, which then attract immunity cells at the site of infection [21, 36].

T lymphocytes CD8+ had no role in controlling the infection and Mtb disease. An activity against Mtb is conceivable considering that T lymphocytes CD8+ recognize Mtb antigens through class I molecules of the major histocompatibility complex (MHC), and produce IL-2, IFN-γ and TNF-α, which have a well-known role in controlling Mtb. This direct cell-to-cell contact determines the apoptosis of the Mtb- infected cell (especially macrophages) depriving Mtb from its natural growth environment and at the same time reducing its viability by unknown mechanism [37]. On the other hand, lymphocytes CD8+ produce IL-10 and TGF-β which instead favor the development of the Mtb infection.

4. Host-directed therapy for tuberculosis

The effectiveness of anti-TB are also influenced by the host immune response due to the interaction of anti-TB. Immuno-modulators' adjunctive therapy that enhance TB might able to shorten treatment durations and improve TB outcomes [38, 39]. To identify new host-directed therapy (HDT) for TB patients is WHO's priority for TB management. Nowadays, Host-directed therapy (HDT) provides a largely unexploited approach as adjunctive anti-TB therapy. Firstly, HDT may impair Mtb replication and survival by disrupting Mtb manipulation of macrophage pathways, thus rendering the bacteria more sensitive to host defenses. The current search for novel therapeutics has focused on the use of repurposed drugs aimed at optimizing the host's response against the mycobacterium [40]. HDT has been proposed as adjuvant therapy for TB infection to improve the efficacy of current treatment outcomes. One possible solution to antibiotic resistance and non-replicating bacterial death problem is targeting the host instead of the pathogen.

Several studies about corticosteroids, TNF blockers, thalidomide, and non-steroidal anti-inflammatory (NSAIDs) have been conducted to determine the function of these immunomodulatory agents as an adjunct of OAT therapy [39, 41]. One of HDT mechanism is autophagy due to its ability in inhibiting the TB infection process [39, 41]. The process of activating autophagy from formation to maturation and then fusion with lysosomes for phagolysosome or autophagy processes requires many activators and protein (ATGs), one of the proteins representing phagolysosome or autophagy is MAP1LC3B/ATG8.

5. Mechanism of action of Metformin as candidate for host-directed therapy in patients with diabetes mellitus: tuberculosis coinfection

Metformin (MET) is a Food and Drug Administration (FDA)-approved drug, biguanide the oral anti diabetic agent, well-known for its glucose-lowering effect on type 2 diabetes (T2D) individuals [1, 2]. A group of studies have reported the potential role of MET as an adjunctive therapy for TB [32, 42, 43]. However, the exact mechanism of how MET modulates the cellular interaction between Mtb and macrophages is not well known. Therefore, we pursued to amalgamate the evidence base on MET as an adjunctive therapy for TB infection using a scoping study methodology to identify gaps to be attained in future research.

Metformin (MET) is the most commonly prescribed drug for type 2 diabetes mellitus. MET through in silico studies, in vitro studies and in vivo studies using animal models, expressed as important role for anti-tuberculosis through immunomodulatory mechanism [42–44], as it is seen in **Figure 5**.

Metformin hydrochloride (MET), recently known has possibilities of utilizing as a combination drug with existing antibiotics for TB therapy [15, 44] and by an extensive in vitro study, MET was reported controlling the growth of drug-resistant Mtb strains via production of mitochondrial reactive oxygen species and facilitates phagosome-lysosome fusion [3, 42]. Thus, MET is known as one of highly potential HDT due to target autophagy by AMPK activation or known as mTOR inhibitor [42, 43].

Moreover, MET is not metabolized by P450 enzymes [1, 2, 45], thus it has no interaction with rifampicin that could decrease the therapy efficacy. However, interaction MET and Rifampicin increases the expression of organic cation transporter (OCT1) and hepatic uptake of metformin, leading to an enhanced glucose lowering [46, 47]. MET is also expected enhanced Isoniazid (INH) efficacy due to SOD activity [48]. INH a pro-drug, its activation is requiring an interaction with Kat-G produced by *Mtb* [1, 2]. Kat-G activation also produces oxidative stress – reactive oxygen species (ROS), namely H_2O_2 and alkyl hydro-peroxides. ROS is neutralized by an antioxidant, superoxide dismutase (SOD). It assumed that SOD contributes to the INH-induced bactericidal effects [32].

5.1 Metformin dan superoxide dismutase (SOD)

Superoxide Dismutase (SOD) is an enzyme produced by the host antioxidant defense system. Increased reactive oxygen species (ROS) as respiratory burst in TB infection results in macrophage phagocytosis process against Mtb. Massive production of ROS also associated with Th1 overactivation, macrophage activity inhibition, and tissue damage. Hyperglycaemia condition could increase ROS production, therefore SOD levels could also increase in DM patients [49]. KatG gene activates INH from pro-drug to active drug. Apparently, SOD contributes during

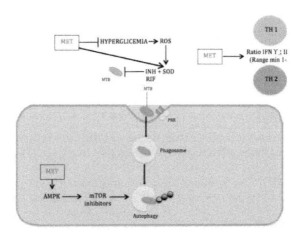

Figure 5.
Mechanism of action Metformin as adjuvant therapy for DM-TB coinfection [32].

this mechanism, higher SOD related to better of INH's in inhibiting Mtb [48]. MET has ability in improving SOD level during inflammation [50, 51]. Based on this, the addition of MET provides synergism effects to increase the effectiveness of INH in treating TB infection. MET also has a synergistic effect with RIF through increasing the expression of organic cation transporter (OCT)-1. The OCT-1 expression plays a role in inhibiting transcription Mtb [9, 44]. Moreover, target of glycemic level for DM-TB patients is also need to be adjusted, therefore synchronized with SOD production [15].

5.2 Metformin induced autophagy

Mtb has an escape mechanism through inhibition of host macrophage cells' autophagy [20, 38]. Improving the autophagia process will improve anti-TB in eliminating Mtb. MET activates Adeno Monophosphate Kinase (AMPK) and subsequent phosphorylation of unc-51-like kinase 1 (ULK1) [52], then AMPK works as mTOR inhibitor and enhances autophagy [37, 39, 42, 43]. Therefore, MET from pharmacodynamics aspect has no effect to Mtb but works on host immune regulation [6, 15].

5.3 Metformin, *interferon gamma* (IFN-γ), *interleukin* (IL)-10 and its ratio

In chronic TB infection, IFN-γ level increases as the body cellular immune response. Currently, IFN-release assay (IGRA) is used as a diagnostic tool for latent TB infection and as an indicator of therapeutic success in active TB infectionf [26, 53, 54]. IL-10 is a negative feedback regulator on the immune response produced by Th2 to inhibit excessive production of pro-inflammatory cytokines. IL-10 barriers the macrophage function, due to suppression of MHC class II molecules and reduces co-stimulator expression [55–57].

MET associated AMPK activation, through thioredoxin-interacting protein (TXNIP) decreases activation of inflammatory mediators and transcription factors, including NF kappa B which encodes proinflammatory mediators [58, 59]. In addition, in intracellular infections such TB MET through AMPK is also stimulated macrophage autophagy [15, 52], therefore MET accelerates Mtb elimination process without excessive inflammatory processes that can damage the tissue [22].

6. Side effects of Metformin that might occur

Gastrointestinal disorders (anorexia, nausea, vomiting and diarrhea) is one of the most common MET's side effect. Impaired absorption of vitamin B_{12}, impaired liver and or kidney function or in elderly people [1, 2]. Increased levels of lactate or known as Metformin-associated lactoacidosis (MALA) although the occurrence is low, must still be prevented. MALA is a life-threatening event. However, in Diabetes Tuberculosis coinfection patients, MALA could be prevented by determining patients criterias, including: 1) has minimal - moderate advaced pulmonary lesions in X-ray chest examination; 2) has oxygen saturation has at least above 92%; 3) has normal liver function (SGOT, SGPT) and normal kidney function (BUN, SK). Providing consultation, information and education related to the symptoms of lacto-acidosis is also needed during MET additional therapy. MET may increase lactate but rarely increase the risk of DM-TB coinfection patients experience MALA [7]. Therefore, MET is relatively safe to use for DM-TB coinfection patients [32].

Abbreviations

TB	Tuberculosis
MET	Metformin
Mtb	*Mycobacterium tuberculosis*
HDT	Host-directed therapy
INH	Isoniazid
DCs	Dendritic cells
IL	Interleukin
INF	Interferon

Author details

Bernadette Dian Novita[1*], Ari Christy Mulyono[2] and Ferdinand Erwin[3]

1 Faculty of Medicine, Department of Pharmacology and Therapy, Widya Mandala Surabaya Catholic University, Indonesia

2 Faculty of Medicine, Department of Internal Medicine, Widya Mandala Surabaya Catholic University, Indonesia

3 Student of Internship Program, Faculty of Medicine, Widya Mandala Surabaya Catholic University, Indonesia

*Address all correspondence to: novita@ukwms.ac.id

IntechOpen

References

[1] Katzung, B. G. B. G. B. G., Mastres, S. B. & Trevor, A. J. *Basic & Clinical Pharmacology*. *Basic and Clinical Pharmacology* (Mc Graw Hill Education (Asia), 2018).

[2] Brunton, L., Hilal-Dandan, R. & Kollman, B. *Goodman & Gilman's The Pharmacological Basis of Therapeutic*. (Mc Graw Hill, 2018). doi:10.4324/9780203813034.

[3] Scarpello, J. H. B. & Howlett, H. C. S. Metformin therapy and clinical uses. Diab. Vasc. Dis. Res. 5, 157-167 (2008).

[4] Li Gonga, Srijib Goswamic, Kathleen M. Giacominic, Russ B. Altmana, b, and T. E. K. Metformin pathways: pharmacokinetics and pharmacodynamics. *Pharmacogenet Genomics* 22, 820-827 (2013).

[5] Lalau, J.-D. Lactic Acidosis Induced by Metformin Incidence , Management and Prevention. *Drug Saf.* 33, 727-740 (2010).

[6] Hur, K. Y. & Lee, M.-S. New mechanisms of metformin action. *J. Diabetes Investig.* 4, n/a-n/a (2015).

[7] Novita, B. D., Pranoto, A., Wuryani, Soediono, E. I. & Mertaniasih, N. M. A case risk study of lactic acidosis risk by metformin use in type 2 diabetes mellitus tuberculosis coinfection patients. *Indian J. Tuberc.* 65, 252-256 (2017).

[8] Brunton, L., Chapner, B. & Knollmann, B. *The Pharmacological Basis of Therapeutics-Goodman & Gillman-Ed*. (Mc Graw Hill Medical, 2011).

[9] Bachmakov, I., Glaeser, H., Fromm, M. F. & König, J. Interaction of oral antidiabetic drugs with hepatic uptake transporters: focus on organic anion transporting polypeptides and organic cation transporter 1. Diabetes 57, 1463-1469 (2008).

[10] Ito, S. *et al.* Competitive inhibition of the luminal efflux by multidrug and toxin extrusions, but not basolateral uptake by organic cation transporter 2, is the likely mechanism underlying the pharmacokinetic drug-drug interactions caused by cimetidine in the kidney. J. Pharmacol. Exp. Ther. 340, 393-403 (2012).

[11] Almeida Da Silva, P. E. A. & Palomino, J. C. Molecular basis and mechanisms of drug resistance in *Mycobacterium tuberculosis*: classical and new drugs. *J. Antimicrob. Chemother.* 66, 1417-30 (2011).

[12] Kumar Nathella, P. & Babu, S. Influence of diabetes mellitus on immunity to human tuberculosis. Immunology 152, 13-24 (2017).

[13] Girardi, E. *et al.* The global dynamics of diabetes and tuberculosis : the impact of migration and policy implications. Int. J. Infect. Dis. 56, 45-53 (2017).

[14] Ogbera, A. O. *et al.* Clinical profile of diabetes mellitus in tuberculosis. BMJ Open Diabetes Res Care 3, e000112 (2015).

[15] Novita, B. D., Ali, M., Pranoto, A., Soediono, E. I. & Mertaniasih, N. M. Metformin induced autophagy in diabetes mellitus – Tuberculosis co-infection patients: A case study. Indian J. Tuberc. 66, 64-69 (2019).

[16] Baghaei, P. *et al.* Impact of diabetes mellitus on tuberculosis drug resistance in new cases of tuberculosis. J. Glob. Antimicrob. Resist. 4, 1-4 (2016).

[17] Nader, L. A., Mattos, A. A. De & Picon, P. D. Hepatotoxicity due to rifampicin , isoniazid and pyrazinamide

in patients with tuberculosis : Is anti-HCV a risk factor ? Ann. Hepatol. **9**, 70-74 (2010).

[18] Sekiguchi, J. *et al.* Detection of multidrug resistance in Mycobacterium tuberculosis. J. Clin. Microbiol. **45**, 179-192 (2007).

[19] Clemens, D. L. *et al.* Targeted intracellular delivery of antituberculosis drugs to Mycobacterium tuberculosis-infected macrophages via functionalized mesoporous silica nanoparticles. Antimicrob. Agents Chemother. **56**, 2535-2545 (2012).

[20] Ernst, J. D. The immunological life cycle of tuberculosis. Nat. Rev. Immunol. **12**, 581-591 (2012).

[21] de Martino, M., Lodi, L., Galli, L. & Chiappini, E. Immune Response to Mycobacterium tuberculosis: A Narrative Review. Front. Pediatr. **7**, 1-8 (2019).

[22] Novita, B. D., Soediono, E. I. & Nugraha, J. Metformin associated inflammation levels regulation in type 2 diabetes mellitus-tuberculosis coinfection patients – A case report. Indian J. Tuberc. **65**, 345-349 (2018).

[23] Das, S. *et al.* Immune subversion by Mycobacterium tuberculosis through CCR5 mediated signaling: Involvement of IL-10. PLoS One **9**, 1-11 (2014).

[24] Lin, C. *et al.* IFN- g Induces Mimic Extracellular Trap. J. Interf. Cytokine Res. **36**, 1-13 (2015).

[25] Lin, C. *et al.* Escape from IFN- γ -dependent immunosurveillance in tumorigenesis. J. Biomed. Sci. **24**, 1-9 (2017).

[26] Chee, C. B. E. *et al.* Tuberculosis treatment effect on T-cell interferon-gamma responses to Mycobacterium tuberculosis-specific antigens. Eur. Respir. J. **36**, 355-361 (2010).

[27] Novita, B. D., Pranoto, A., Wuryani, Soediono, E. I. & Mertaniasih, N. M. A Case Risk-Study of Lactic Acidosis Risk in Metformin Use in Type 2 Diabetes Mellitus Tuberculosis co-Infection Patients. *Indian J. Tuberc.* (2017) doi:10.1016/j.ijtb.2017.05.008.

[28] Cavalcanti, Y. V. N., Brelaz, M. C. A., Neves, J. K. D. A. L., Ferraz, J. C. & Pereira, V. R. A. Role of TNF-alpha, IFN-gamma, and IL-10 in the development of pulmonary tuberculosis. *Pulm. Med.* **2012**, (2012).

[29] Abbas, A. K. & Lichtman, A. *Cellular and Molecular Immunology.* (Saunders, 2012).

[30] Dobrian, a D. *et al.* Dipeptidyl peptidase IV inhibitor sitagliptin reduces local inflammation in adipose tissue and in pancreatic islets of obese mice. *Am. J. Physiol. Endocrinol. Metab.* **300**, E410-21 (2011).

[31] Clark, I., Atwood, C., Bowen, R., Paz-filho, G. & Vissel, B. Tumor Necrosis Factor-Induced Cerebral Insulin Resistance in Alzheimer' s Disease Links Numerous Treatment Rationales. Pharmacol. Rev. **64**, 1004-1026 (2012).

[32] Novita, B. D. Metformin: A review of its potential as enhancer for anti tuberculosis efficacy in diabetes mellitus-tuberculosis coinfection patients. Indian J. Tuberc. **66**, 294-298 (2019).

[33] Singhal, J. *et al.* Suppression of dendritic cell-mediated responses by genes in calcium and cysteine protease pathways during Mycobacterium tuberculosis infection. J. Biol. Chem. **287**, 11108-11121 (2012).

[34] Restrepo, B. I. *et al.* Tuberculosis in poorly controlled type 2 diabetes: altered cytokine expression in peripheral white blood cells. Clin. Infect. Dis. **47**, 634-641 (2008).

[35] Welin, A. Survival strategies of *Mycobacterium tuberculosis* inside the human macrophage. (Linkoping University, 2011).

[36] Feng, W. X. *et al.* CCL2-2518 (A/G) polymorphisms and tuberculosis susceptibility: A meta-analysis. Int. J. Tuberc. Lung Dis. **16**, 150-156 (2012).

[37] Uhlin, M., Andersson, J., Zumla, A. & Maeurer, M. Adjunct Immunotherapies for Tuberculosis. J. Infect. Dis. **205**, 325-334 (2012).

[38] Caire-Brändli, I. *et al.* Reversible lipid accumulation and associated division arrest of Mycobacterium avium in lipoprotein-induced foamy macrophages may resemble key events during latency and reactivation of tuberculosis. Infect. Immun. **82**, 476-490 (2014).

[39] Wallis, R. S. & Hafner, R. Advancing host-directed therapy for tuberculosis. Nature Reviews Immunology vol. 15 255-263 (2015).

[40] Rakshit, S. *et al.* Circulating Mycobacterium tuberculosis DosR latency antigen-specific, polyfunctional, regulatory IL10+ Th17 CD4 T-cells differentiate latent from active tuberculosis. Sci. Rep. 7, 1-15 (2017).

[41] Hawn, T. R., Matheson, A. I. & Maley, S. N. Host-Directed Therapeutics for Tuberculosis : Can We Harness the Host ? Microbiol. Mol. Biol. Rev. 77, 608-627 (2013).

[42] Singhal, A. *et al.* Metformin as adjunct antituberculosis therapy. *Sci. Transl. Med.* **6**, 263ra159-263ra159 (2014).

[43] Restrepo, B. I. Metformin: Candidate host-directed therapy for tuberculosis in diabetes and non-diabetes patients. Tuberculosis **101**, S69–S72 (2016).

[44] Vashisht, R. & Brahmachari, S. K. Metformin as a potential combination therapy with existing front-line antibiotics for Tuberculosis. J. Transl. Med. **13**, 1-3 (2015).

[45] Madiraju, A. K. *et al.* Metformin suppresses gluconeogenesis by inhibiting mitochondrial glycerophosphate dehydrogenase. Nature **510**, 542-546 (2014).

[46] Thee, S. *et al.* Pharmacokinetics of isoniazid, rifampin, and pyrazinamide in children younger than two years of age with tuberculosis: evidence for implementation of revised World Health Organization recommendations. Antimicrob. Agents Chemother. **55**, 5560-5567 (2011).

[47] Sousa, M., Pozniak, A. & Boffito, M. Pharmacokinetics and pharmacodynamics of drug interactions involving rifampicin, rifabutin and antimalarial drugs. J. Antimicrob. Chemother. **62**, 872-878 (2008).

[48] Palanisamy, N. & Manian, S. Protective effects of Asparagus racemosus on oxidative damage in isoniazid-induced hepatotoxic rats: an in vivo study. Toxicol. Ind. Health **28**, 238-244 (2012).

[49] Omori, K. *et al.* Priming of neutrophil oxidative burst in diabetes requires preassembly of the NADPH oxidase. J. Leukoc. Biol. **84**, 292-301 (2008).

[50] Yilmaz, B. *et al.* Metformin regresses endometriotic implants in rats by improving implant levels of superoxide dismutase, vascular endothelial growth factor, tissue inhibitor of metalloproteinase-2, and matrix metalloproteinase-9. *Am. J. Obstet. Gynecol.* **202**, 368.e1-8 (2010).

[51] Hink, J., Thom, S. R., Simonsen, U., Rubin, I. & Jansen, E. Vascular reactivity and endothelial NOS activity

in rat thoracic aorta during and after hyperbaric oxygen exposure. Am. J. Physiol. Heart Circ. Physiol. **291**, H1988-H1998 (2006).

[52] Zhuang, Y. & Miskimins, W. K. Metformin induces both caspase-dependent and poly(ADP-ribose) polymerase-dependent cell death in breast cancer cells. Mol. Cancer Res. **9**, 603-615 (2011).

[53] Lange, C., Pai, M., Drobniewski, F. & Migliori, G. B. Interferon-gamma release assays for the diagnosis of active tuberculosis: sensible or silly? Eur. Respir. J. **33**, 1250-1253 (2009).

[54] Matsushita, I. *et al.* Dynamics of immune parameters during the treatment of active tuberculosis showing negative interferon gamma response at the time of diagnosis. Int. J. Infect. Dis. **40**, 39-44 (2015).

[55] Gaultier, A. *et al.* Regulation of tumor necrosis factor receptor-1 and the IKK-NF-kappaB pathway by LDL receptor-related protein explains the antiinflammatory activity of this receptor. Blood **111**, 5316-5325 (2008).

[56] Yuhas, Y., Berent, E., Cohen, R. & Ashkenazi, S. Roles of NF-kappaB activation and peroxisome proliferator-activated receptor gamma inhibition in the effect of rifampin on inducible nitric oxide synthase transcription in human lung epithelial cells. Antimicrob. Agents Chemother. **53**, 1539-1545 (2009).

[57] Kresno, S. B. *Imunologi : Diagnosis dan Prosedur Laboratorium*. (Badan Penerbit Fakultas Kedokteran Universitas Indonesia, 2013).

[58] Salminen, A., Hyttinen, J. M. T. & Kaarniranta, K. AMP-activated protein kinase inhibits NF-κB signaling and inflammation: impact on healthspan and lifespan. J. Mol. Med. (Berl). **89**, 667-76 (2011).

[59] Wan, X. *et al.* 5'-AMP-activated protein kinase-activating transcription factor 1 cascade modulates human monocyte-derived macrophages to atheroprotective functions in response to heme or metformin. Arterioscler. Thromb. Vasc. Biol. **33**, 2470-2480 (2013).

Lightning Source UK Ltd.
Milton Keynes UK
UKHW051146120223
416791UK00010B/249